T0316693

Curbside Consultation
in Pediatric Asthma

49 Clinical Questions

Curbside Consultation in Pediatrics
SERIES

SERIES EDITOR, LISA B. ZAOUTIS

Curbside Consultation
in Pediatric Asthma

49 Clinical Questions

EDITOR

Aaron S. Chidekel, MD
Associate Professor of Pediatrics
Jefferson Medical College of Thomas Jefferson University
Chief, Division of Pulmonology
Nemours at the Alfred I. duPont Hospital for Children
Wilmington, Delaware

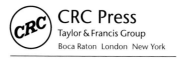

CRC Press
Taylor & Francis Group
Boca Raton London New York

CRC Press is an imprint of the
Taylor & Francis Group, an **informa** business

First published 2012 by SLACK Incorporated

Published 2024 by CRC Press
2385 NW Executive Center Drive, Suite 320, Boca Raton FL 33431

and by CRC Press
4 Park Square, Milton Park, Abingdon, Oxon, OX14 4RN

CRC Press is an imprint of Taylor & Francis Group, LLC

Library of Congress Cataloging-in-Publication Data

Curbside consultation in pediatric asthma : 49 clinical questions / editor, Aaron Chidekel.
    p. ; cm. -- (Curbside consultation in pediatrics series)
  Pediatric asthma
  Includes bibliographical references and index.
  ISBN 978-1-55642-987-3 (alk. paper)
  I. Chidekel, Aaron. II. Title: Pediatric asthma. III. Series: Curbside consultation in pediatrics series.
  [DNLM: 1. Asthma--diagnosis. 2. Asthma--therapy. 3. Child. WF 553]
  LC classification not assigned
  618.92′238--dc23
                          2012005903

ISBN: 9781556429873 (pbk)
ISBN: 9781003523611 (ebk)

DOI: 10.1201/9781003523611

Dedication

For Stacy and the other 3 "C's."

For my parents who first instilled in me a love of books.

Contents

Acknowledgments

I acknowledge and thank my most important mentors: Those who taught me how to ask questions including Gabriel G. Haddad, MD, and those who taught me how to find the answers needed by my patients, including Thomas F. Dolan Jr, MD and Marie E. Egan, MD. I also thank my friend and colleague Kate Cronan, MD for her thorough and thoughtful review of the manuscript.

About the Editor

Aaron S. Chidekel, MD received his medical degree from Brown University in Providence, Rhode Island. He completed his internship and residency in general pediatrics at Yale-New Haven Hospital. He completed fellowship training in pediatric respiratory medicine in the Section of Respiratory Medicine at the Yale University School of Medicine. After completing his training, Dr. Chidekel moved to the Nemours at the Alfred I. duPont Hospital for Children in Wilmington, Delaware. He is currently Chief of the Division of Pulmonology at the Alfred I. duPont Hospital for Children and Director of the Sleep Medicine and Cystic Fibrosis Programs as well. He is an Associate Professor of Pediatrics at the Jefferson Medical College of Thomas Jefferson University. Dr. Chidekel has authored numerous scientific papers and abstracts in various aspects of clinical and basic research related to pediatric pulmonary medicine. He has contributed chapters to several textbooks and has served as a reviewer for many prestigious journals as well. He is a fellow in the American Academy of Pediatrics and has been active as an officer and board member of the Delaware Chapter, and is a member of the American Thoracic Society and the American Academy of Sleep Medicine.

Contributing Authors

Alia Bazzy-Asaad, MD (Questions 20 & 22)
Associate Professor of Pediatrics
Chief, Section of Pediatric Respiratory
  Medicine
Department of Pediatrics
Yale University School of Medicine
New Haven, Connecticut

*Jonathan E. Bennett, MD (Questions 32, 33,
  34, & 35)*
Associate Professor of Pediatrics
Jefferson Medical College
Nemours at the Alfred I. duPont Hospital
  for Children
Division of Emergency Medicine
Wilmington, Delaware

Anita Bhandari, MD (Questions 9 & 26)
Assistant Professor of Pediatrics
University of Connecticut School of
  Medicine
Director, Sickle Cell Pulmonary Program
Director, Chronic Infant Lung Disease
  (ChILD) Program
Director, Pediatric Pulmonology
  Fellowship
Attending Physician
Division of Pediatric Pulmonology
Connecticut Children's Medical Center
Hartford, Connecticut

Brad Bley, DO, CSCS (Questions 24 & 31)
Primary Care Sports Medicine
Internal Medicine/Pediatrics
Delaware Orthopaedic Specialists
Newark, Delaware

Lisa Forbes, MD (Questions 10, 11, & 12)
Division of Allergy and Immunology
Children's Hospital of Philadelphia
Philadelphia, Pennsylvania

David E. Geller, MD (Question 14)
Associate Professor of Pediatrics
College of Medicine
Florida State University
Tallahassee, Florida

Natalie M. Hayes, DO (Questions 8, 13, & 43)
Assistant Professor of Pediatrics
Wake Forest University School of Medicine
Department of Pediatrics
Wake Forest Baptist Health
Winston-Salem, North Carolina

Robert A. Heinle, MD (Questions 1, 2, 3, 4, & 5)
Assistant Professor of Pediatrics and
  Internal Medicine
Jefferson Medical College of
  Thomas Jefferson University
Division of Pulmonology
Nemours at the Alfred I. duPont Hospital
  for Children
Wilmington, Delaware

Katherine A. King, MD (Questions 6 & 7)
Associate Professor in Clinical Pediatrics
Thomas Jefferson University
School of Medicine
Nemours at the Alfred I. duPont Hospital
  for Children
Wilmington, Delaware

*Joel D. Klein, MD, FAAP (Questions 17, 18,
  & 44)*
Professor of Pediatrics
Jefferson Medical College
Philadelphia, Pennsylvania
Division of Infectious Diseases
Nemours at the Alfred I. duPont Hospital
  for Children
Wilmington, Delaware

Jennifer LeComte, DO (Questions 17, 18, & 44)
Internal Medicine-Pediatrics
Pediatric Chief Resident
Nemours at the Alfred I. duPont Hospital
    for Children
Wilmington, Delaware

Holger Link, MD (Question 25)
Clinical Associate Professor
Oregon Health & Science University
Department of Pediatrics
Division of Pediatric Pulmonology
Doernbecher Children's Hospital
Portland, Oregon

Stephen J. McGeady, MD (Questions 15, 19, & 45)
Allergy, Asthma and Immunology
    Specialist
Director, Allergy & Immunology
    Fellowship program
Nemours at the Alfred I. duPont Hospital
    for Children
Division of Allergy, Asthma
    & Immunology
Wilmington, Delaware

Sheela Raikar, MD (Question 16)
Pediatric Gastroenterology Fellow
Thomas Jefferson University
Nemours at the Alfred I. duPont Hospital
    for Children
Wilmington, Delaware

Gabriela Ramirez-Garnica, PhD, MPH (Question 48)
Nemours Children's Clinic
Orlando, Florida

Amy Renwick, MD (Questions 21 & 27)
Assistant Professor of Pediatrics
Jefferson Medical College
Philadelphia, Pennsylvania
Director of Primary and
    Consultative Pediatrics
Nemours at the Alfred I. duPont Hospital
    for Children
Wilmington, Delaware

Julie Ryu, MD (Question 46)
Associate Clinical Professor of Pediatrics
University of California, San Diego
Department of Pediatrics, Division of
    Respiratory Medicine
Rady Children's Hospital-San Diego
San Diego, California

Jonathan M. Spergel, MD, PhD (Questions 10, 11, & 12)
Associate Professor of Pediatrics
The Children's Hospital of Philadelphia
Division of Allergy and Immunology
Perelman School of Medicine
University of Pennsylvania
Philadelphia, Pennsylvania

Concettina (Tina) Tolomeo DNP, APRN, FNP-BC, AE-C (Questions 28, 38, 39, 40, & 47)
Nurse Practitioner
Director of Program Development
Yale University School of Medicine
Section of Pediatric Respiratory Medicine
New Haven, Connecticut

Daniel J. Weiner, MD (Questions 41 & 42)
Division of Pulmonary Medicine
Co-Director, Antonio J. & Janet Palumbo
    Cystic Fibrosis Center
Medical Director, Pulmonary Function
    Laboratory
Children's Hospital of Pittsburgh of UPMC
Pittsburgh, Pennsylvania

Lisa B. Zaoutis, MD (Question 36)
Assistant Professor of Pediatrics
The Perelman School of Medicine at
    the University of Pennsylvania
Director, Pediatric Residency Program
The Children's Hospital of Philadelphia
Philadelphia, Pennsylvania

Preface

Pediatric asthma is a topic of great importance that spans many areas of medical practice from general pediatrics to the subspecialties of pediatric allergy and immunology and pulmonology. Collaborating providers in nursing and respiratory care also have critically important roles in the management, testing, and education of children and families affected by this most common of all pediatric chronic diseases. In selecting the most pertinent issues in pediatric asthma for presentation in *Curbside Consultation in Pediatric Asthma: 49 Clinical Questions*, topics were prioritized with the intention of reflecting the multidisciplinary nature of asthma care and with the intention of reaching out to this diverse team of providers.

Asthma is also a diverse subject. It is a subject that perhaps better lends itself to 49 entire textbooks rather than one text with 49 concise questions and answers! Herein is the value and utility of *Curbside Consultation in Pediatric Asthma: 49 Clinical Questions*. It will introduce the reader to the breadth of the topic and hit the critical subjects in a concise and "user-friendly" format that is patient and practitioner focused. It can serve as a quick reference or roadmap, just like stopping a colleague in the hallway can provide quick and relevant insights that can be implemented quickly and efficiently.

In formulating the individual sections or questions and answers in *Curbside Consultation in Pediatric Asthma: 49 Clinical Questions*, my career as a consultant pulmonologist and as a curbside consultant in particular influenced the goals and objectives for the project. A helpful and collegial curbside consult needs to be handled with efficiency from an expert perspective and be soundly evidence based. These 3 characteristics make a curbside consult helpful and it is my hope that each of the chapters in the book fulfills this mandate. A curbside consult is not meant to be exhaustive, but rather serve a dual purpose to provide a practical solution or answer to the question at hand and to serve as a springboard for further exploration of the medical literature for the person asking the question.

Curbside Consultation in Pediatric Asthma: 49 Clinical Questions should serve as a useful resource for the student just learning about asthma or the seasoned practitioner in need of a quick clinical reference or even a refresher on the topic of pediatric asthma. I hope you enjoy it and would stop me in the hallway again for another curbside on this or any other clinical topic that is puzzling you!

Aaron S. Chidekel, MD

Foreword

While there are several comprehensive textbooks on pediatric respiratory medicine that are well worth owning and having on the shelves of our offices, there are very few texts focusing solely on pediatric asthma. *Curbside Consultation in Pediatric Asthma: 49 Clinical Questions* will fill this gap in our office shelves nicely. It is approachable for the generalist, comprehensive for the specialist, and succinct enough for anyone who is a busy clinician. While it is clearly a difficult task to achieve all 3 of those goals, *Curbside Consultation in Pediatric Asthma: 49 Clinical Questions* will provide the reader with a broad and yet detailed overview of this important topic.

Curbside Consultation in Pediatric Asthma: 49 Clinical Questions is clearly written for the primary care physician who is busy in the trenches addressing the often complicated needs of children with asthma. It is also ideal for the trainees who are "growing" in the field and who would like to have rapid access to practical answers on the inpatient ward, in the emergency department, and in the outpatient clinic. *Curbside Consultation in Pediatric Asthma: 49 Clinical Questions* also offers suggestions for further reading that is up-to-date and practical. Another terrific aspect of this book is that all of the contributors are actively seeing patients. These authors are the generalists and subspecialists who should be giving such practical answers to their colleagues' questions, whether they are primary care physicians, subspecialists, trainees or students.

While asthma care is clearly a team effort, a major part of the care of these children will be given in increasing proportion by the primary care physician. Another important aim of asthma treatment is to prevent admissions to the hospital and establish effective long-term management plans for all patients. Finally, when necessary, the primary care physician and the asthma specialist must "team up" to provide effective intervention for the most complicated and vulnerable asthmatic children. One question and chapter at a time, *Curbside Consultation in Pediatric Asthma: 49 Clinical Questions* will provide an important learning resource about the most recent advances in asthma care, the type of education that patients need, the asthma plan to follow, and what to constantly look for in order to intervene earlier rather than later. In addition to all of this, there are also chapters and questions dedicated to the management of the pediatric asthma patient when in the hospital, the emergency department, or even in your office.

I applaud the effort taken to put this comprehensive and succinct book together. *Curbside Consultation in Pediatric Asthma: 49 Clinical Questions,* with its various chapters and questions, will be a useful resource for all members of the asthma care team whether they are based in the hospital, the outpatient department, or in the private office.

Gabriel G. Haddad, MD
Chair, Department of Pediatrics
University of California, San Diego
La Jolla, California

SECTION I

ASTHMA EPIDEMIOLOGY

How Big of a Problem
Is Childhood Asthma?

Robert A. Heinle, MD

Asthma is a chronic respiratory disease associated with intermittent episodes of coughing, wheezing, chest tightness, and respiratory distress. These episodes may be extremely alarming to children as well as their families. In addition to these more acute episodes, asthma may result in frequent symptoms which can lead to activity limitation, sleep disruption, and school absenteeism. These asthma symptoms are chronic and troublesome and may be present in children who have never required emergency care for their illness. Another common feature of childhood asthma is prolonged and/or recurrent respiratory infection with protracted symptoms of coughing and wheezing. The complaint of recurrent pneumonia or lower respiratory tract infections with wheezing is particularly common and should also alert the physician to the possibility of asthma.

Despite ongoing advances in our understanding of the pathophysiology and treatment of asthma, it remains a significant cause of morbidity and mortality in children. For reasons that remain unclear, the prevalence of asthma in children increased steadily over 15 years between 1980 and 1995. During this time, the prevalence of asthma nearly doubled (Figure 1-1). In 1997, the National Health Interview Survey was redesigned with expanded asthma definitions; however, review of the prevalence before and after this change showed that asthma remained at a similar high level. Current asthma prevalence has continued to climb steadily during the past decade as well. In 2005, pediatric asthma prevalence was estimated at nearly 6 million children (8.9%). In 2007, the prevalence had increased to 9.1%, and the most recent data from 2009 estimate an asthma prevalence of 9.6% (7.1 million children). In the National Health Interview Survey, there were an additional 3 million children who had a history of asthma previously (but not currently), bringing the total prevalence of children between the ages of 0 and 17 with a "history of asthma" to 12.7%. These sobering statistics make asthma the most common chronic lung disease of childhood, and it is clear that a significant asthma epidemic continues unabated in the United States.

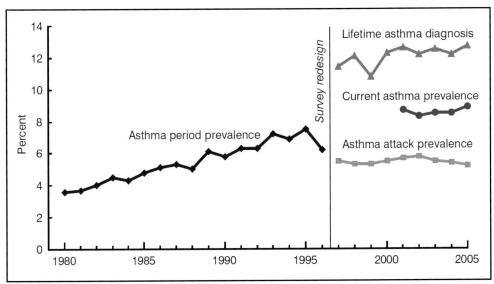

Figure 1-1. Asthma prevalence among children 0 to 17 years of age for measures of asthma prevalence available in each year, United States, 1980–2005. (Adapted from data from the Centers for Disease Control/National Center for Health Statistics, National Health Interview Survey.)

The care of this significant number of asthmatic patients has an enormous impact on medical resource utilization. In the ambulatory setting, there has been a significant increase in physician office and outpatient hospital visits for asthma despite a plateau in the prevalence of asthma. This is likely multifactorial, including increased public awareness of asthma symptoms and severity, the need to establish severity and control, and increased focus on early interventions during acute exacerbations. In 2004, nearly 2.5% of all physician outpatient visits for children were due to asthma (6.5 million visits).

Asthma exacerbations are often managed in the emergency department. Despite the increase in the number of outpatient asthma visits to primary care physician offices, there has been no decrease in the number of emergency department visits. The frequency of emergency department visits has been fairly stable over the previous 15 years. In 2004, asthma exacerbations in children represented 2.8% of all emergency department visits (750,000 visits). While this figure decreased somewhat to 640,000 in 2007, this remains a significant concern because recurrent visits to the emergency department for asthma flares are a risk factor for dying from asthma. In fact, the prevention of emergency department visits is an important clinical and quality outcome goal, indicating that emergency care for asthma episodes should be a routine topic of conversation during regular asthma follow-up care.

Children with asthma exacerbations that are not responsive to outpatient therapy are admitted to the hospital. Hospital admission can be a stressful experience for children and their families and results in further disruption of their lives and activities. Hospitalization rates for asthma have followed prevalence rates for asthma with several years of incline followed by a plateau at recent high levels. Asthma exacerbations accounted for 3% of all hospitalizations of children (nearly 200,000 hospitalizations). At my own institution, asthma is among the most common discharge diagnosis. The average length of stay is approximately 2 days and a significant proportion (~20%) of children with asthma require repeated admissions for the management of their disease.

Rarely, children can die from their asthma. Mortality rates from asthma rose in parallel with the prevalence of asthma through much of the 1980s and 1990s; however, there was a decrease in asthma mortality from 1999 to 2004. In 2004, there continued to be 2.5 asthma deaths per 1 million children (186 deaths total). Of all the available asthma therapies, inhaled corticosteroids have been shown to be protective against asthma mortality in children.

Cumulatively, the 2010 direct cost of the care for asthma in the United States is estimated at $15.6 billion of health care expenditures. An additional $5.1 billion is related to indirect costs associated with morbidity and mortality, for a total of more than $20 billion! There are nonmonetary costs of asthma as well. The 4 million children with 1 asthma attack in the previous year missed a combined total of 12.8 million school days. Asthma causes a significant number of missed work days for the parents of these children in addition to the 10 million missed work days for adults with asthma.

Summary

Despite improved understanding of the pathophysiology of asthma and its treatment, the cost of childhood asthma in terms of money, disability, and lives lost remains high. This combination of medical, psychosocial, and economic factors is often referred to as the "burden" of asthma both to children and society, and reducing this burden remains a critical goal for those of us caring for this common and morbid condition.

Suggested Readings

Akinbami L. The state of childhood asthma, United States, 1980-2005. Advance data from *Vital and Health Statistics, Centers for Disease Control and Prevention*. 2006;381:1-28.

Akinbami LJ, Moorman JE, Garbe PL, Sondik EJ. Status of childhood asthma in the United States, 1980-2007. *Pediatrics*. 2009;123:S131-S145.

National Asthma Education and Prevention Program. *Expert panel report 3 (EPR-3): guidelines for the diagnosis and management of asthma*. Bethesda, MD: National Heart, Lung, and Blood Institute, 2007. NIH publication no. 08-4051.

National Institutes of Health. *National Heart, Lung, and Blood Institute Chartbook on Cardiovascular, Lung, and Blood Diseases*. Washington, DC: U.S. Department of Health & and Human Services; 2009.

WHO IS AT RISK FOR DEVELOPING ASTHMA?

Robert A. Heinle, MD

As our understanding of asthma grows, our appreciation for its complexity has grown as well. Asthma is no longer thought of as a single entity with a single origin, but as a complex spectrum of host and environmental factors that lead to the final common findings of airflow obstruction, bronchial hyper-responsiveness, and underlying airway inflammation. This cascade of genetic and environmental factors manifests as episodes of wheezing, breathlessness, chest tightness, and coughing, particularly at night or in the early morning and can evolve over the life of an individual and vary strikingly over time. These host predispositions and environmental exposures are present at a very early age (Figure 2-1). Host predispositions include genetics, gender, atopy or immunoglobulin-E (IgE) production, airway hyper-responsiveness (AHR), prematurity, and the cytokine response profile. Relevant environmental exposures include allergens, irritants, and infections, and the exposure to these at critical periods during development can have lasting implications that may favor the development of asthma or perhaps protect against its development.

The genetic basis of asthma clearly includes an inherited familial component, but this inheritance does not follow simple Mendelian genetics. There are likely multiple genes in multiple locations of the human genome that impact the predisposition toward asthma, and it is likely that there are other genes that function as modifiers of asthma severity. Additionally, there appear to be genetic influences on IgE production, AHR, and changes in inflammatory regulators (ie, cytokines) that are each independent risk factors for the development of asthma. Identifying these specific genes and their impact on the development and severity of asthma is the subject of ongoing research but remains to be fully defined.

Male gender has a higher association with asthma at young ages than female gender. For adolescents, the association of gender with current asthma equalizes as it transitions to a higher incidence of asthma in adult women. The reason for this change in relative risk over a lifetime remains unclear. There have been investigations into sex hormones

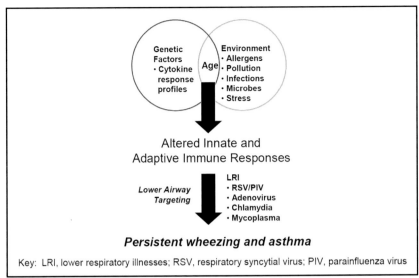

Key: LRI, lower respiratory illnesses; RSV, respiratory syncytial virus; PIV, parainfluenza virus

Figure 2-1. Host factors and environmental exposures. (Adapted from National Asthma Education and Prevention Program. *Expert panel report 3: guidelines for the diagnosis and management of asthma.* Bethesda, MD: National Heart, Lung, and Blood Institute, 2007.)

and pubertal factors, as well as changes in airway caliber relative to vital capacity, but the results are inconsistent and the exact reason for this gender relationship to asthma prevalence remains elusive.

Atopy involves the genetic tendency to develop IgE antibodies in response to the exposure to environmental stimuli or allergens. When IgE is bound to mast cells, it triggers the release of multiple pro-inflammatory signals including histamine and cytokines such as interleukin (IL)-4. These signals are then involved in the development and maintenance of airway inflammation and AHR. There appears to be a direct correlation between IgE level measured in the blood and the presence of AHR. Therefore, IgE may be one of the prominent mediators during acute flares of asthma after exposure to airborne allergens. Approximately 50% of asthma cases are attributable to atopy. Additionally, there is a steroid-sparing effect in patients with severe steroid-dependent asthma by decreasing IgE levels with therapies such as omalizumab, a humanized anti-IgE antibody. This further substantiates the role of atopy and elevated IgE levels as risk factors for asthma.

AHR to inhaled irritants or allergens is a key part of asthma pathophysiology. AHR is the tendency of the airway to react or bronchoconstrict after exposure to a stimulant. Most patients with AHR are asymptomatic at the time of testing, and many do not go on to develop asthma. This suggests that asthma is a subset of AHR. However, having AHR increases the risk of developing asthma by nearly 5 times.

Prematurity defined as gestational age less than 37 weeks is associated with an increased risk of asthma and asthma-like illnesses. This association is stronger for females and infants who required mechanical ventilation to treat lung immaturity associated with prematurity. To quantify the exact increase in asthma risk has been difficult due to conflicting studies. For example, some studies have shown an increased risk of asthma due

Table 2-1
Cytokine Balance Between T-Helper Lymphocytes

Factors Favoring the Th1 Phenotype	*Factors Favoring the Th2 Phenotype*
Presence of older siblings	Widespread use of antibiotics
Early exposure to daycare	Western lifestyle
Tuberculosis, measles, or hepatitis A infection	Urban environment
Rural environment	Diet
	Sensitization to house dust mites and cockroaches

to prematurity as high as 3 to 4 times that seen in the general population. If true, this means that up to 50% of premature infants may go on to develop asthma.

An individual's cytokine response profile may cross both host predispositions and environmental factors. Cytokines are one of the major signaling mechanisms of the immune system and play a significant role in modifying the inflammatory response in asthma. The cytokines released by T-helper 2 (Th2) lymphocytes, such as IL-4, IL-5, and IL-13, promote the increase of IgE levels in the blood, the presence of airway eosinophils, and the development of AHR. The Th2 cytokine profile promotes allergic diseases, in general, including asthma, whereas the T-helper 1 (Th1) cytokine profile is protective (Table 2-1). Environmental exposures and infections can influence the balance between Th1 and Th2 cytokines, thereby increasing or decreasing the risk of asthma.

Allergen sensitization and ongoing exposure is a risk factor for the development of asthma. Some of the most common allergens associated with the development of asthma in children are the house dust mite, cockroaches, and *Alternaria* (a common fungus). Exposure to cat and dog dander has been controversial because some research links animal exposure to increased incidence of asthma and asthma flares, while other studies suggest a protective role of these exposures. The "Hygiene Hypothesis" is being actively investigated to define further the role of various environmental exposures at critical developmental stages in the development of asthma and other allergic diseases.

Some respiratory infections early in life are associated with the development of asthma. Specifically, the risk of developing asthma or asthma-like symptoms even years after a documented respiratory syncytial virus (RSV) infection early in life has been reported to be as high as 40%. Other infectious etiologies now being linked to the development of asthma include para-influenza virus and rhinovirus. However, some infections appear to shift the cytokine profile toward the Th1 profile and may provide a protective effect. This is related to the "Hygiene Hypothesis," which states that early infections (particularly certain bacterial exposure or colonization) may influence the development of atopy in a protective manner by shifting an individual cytokine profile toward a Th1 paradigm and that the increasingly sterile environment in which we live does not allow the shift of cytokines away from those that favor the development allergic diseases and asthma (Th2 paradigm).

Other irritants, such as environmental tobacco smoke (ETS) exposure, have clearly been shown to exacerbate existing asthma, decrease the ability to control asthma consistently, and increase respiratory symptoms. Limiting exposure to toxic ETS is important at any age and is clearly beneficial to all children and not just those with asthma. ETS is one of the most well-studied modifiers of asthma severity.

As our understanding of asthma grows, our appreciation of all the factors that predispose an individual to its development has also grown. These risk factors are the subject of ongoing research and may evolve over time as our understanding of the complicated signaling pathways is further clarified. In the meantime, these risk factors can be discussed with patients and family at the bedside to target those patients at highest risk of developing asthma.

Suggested Readings

Arbes SJ Jr, Gergen PJ, Vaughn B, Zeldin DC. Asthma cases attributable to atopy: results from the Third National Health and Nutrition Examination Survey. *J Allergy Clin Immunol*. 2007;120:1139.

National Asthma Education and Prevention Program. *Expert panel report 3 (EPR-3): guidelines for the diagnosis and management of asthma*. Bethesda, MD: National Heart, Lung, and Blood Institute, 2007. NIH publication no. 08-4051.

Porsbjerg C, von Linstow ML, Ulrik CS, et al. Risk factors for onset of asthma: a 12-year prospective follow-up study. *Chest*. 2006;129:309.

WHICH GROUPS OF CHILDREN ARE MOST IMPACTED BY CHILDHOOD ASTHMA?

Robert A. Heinle, MD

Asthma has been found in children of all ages, of both genders, and in all ethnicities; however, the prevalence of asthma varies throughout life and to varying degrees between gender and ethnicities. Socioeconomic factors are also important, and asthma remains a disease that reflects larger health disparities in the United States. The most common risk factors for asthma continue to involve the complex interplay between familial and genetic influences coupled with infectious and noninfectious environmental exposures at critical developmental periods. Cases of asthma tend to be grouped in families that have a high incidence of atopy, and asthma is common in certain ethnic groups and among socially disadvantaged members of society (see Question 2).

Children may develop asthma at different ages of their life, but the prevalence of asthma tends to increase with age. The overall prevalence of asthma in children 0 to 4 years of age was 6.2% in 2005. This increased to an overall prevalence of 9.3% in children 5 to 10 years of age. Finally, there was a small but continued increase to 10.0% in those children ages 11 to 17 years. This results in an overall prevalence of 9.6% asthma in children younger than age 18. This trend is in contrast to medical resource utilization including outpatient visits, emergency room visits, and hospitalizations, which tend to decrease as children with asthma get older. Thus, despite the lowest prevalence of asthma at the youngest ages (younger than 2 years), there tends to be the highest medical resource utilization (Figure 3-1) among children in this age group.

This inverse relationship of asthma prevalence and medical resource utilization is thought to be multifactorial. There is difficulty differentiating airway inflammation and symptoms due to asthma from airway inflammation due to recurrent viral infections at young ages, and this may delay a formal diagnosis of asthma. However, the tendency of the small airways of young children to become obstructed may result in much more dramatic and severe symptoms during asthma flares that warrant increased urgent medical care. Similarly, viral infections are more frequent in young children. As children get

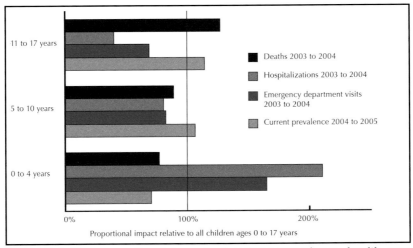

Figure 3-1. The proportional impact of asthma prevalence, health care use, and mortality among children 0 to 17 years of age, by age group, United States, 2003–2005. (Adapted from data from the Centers for Disease Control/National Center for Health Statistics, National Health Interview Survey, National Hospital Ambulatory Medical Care Survey, and the Mortality Component of the National Vital Statistic System.)

older, there is greater confidence in eliciting a history of chronic coughing and wheezing associated with common asthma triggers. There may also be a greater self-awareness of symptoms and enhanced ability to identify asthma flares earlier in their course that may preclude the need for urgent evaluations. On the other hand, adolescents remain a medically underserved population and are notorious for denying, under-reporting, or misperceiving asthma symptoms.

There is a discrepancy between males and females and the impact of asthma in most age groups in childhood. The prevalence and medical resource utilization is slightly higher in boys than in girls from infancy through adolescence. The most recent data from the Centers for Disease Control (CDC) report that the overall asthma prevalence in boys is 11.3%. However, in late adolescence (15 to 17 years of age), the prevalence of asthma in girls (10.5%) exceeds boys (10.1%), and this trend continues into adulthood. There is also a greater use of medical resources in the ambulatory setting by teenage girls than boys, although hospitalization and death rates remain slightly higher in boys. This inverse relationship between utilization of medical resources in the ambulatory setting and asthma-related hospitalization or death is also seen in the racial disparity of asthma.

The impact of race and ethnicity is a complex and fluid interaction of genetics and environment. Prevalence rates of asthma range from the lowest in children of Asian descent to the highest in those children of Puerto Rican ethnicity (Table 3-1). Non-Hispanic Black children also have a strikingly high asthma prevalence of 17% according to the most recently published statistics from the CDC. Table 3-1 also shows the inverse relationship between the number of ambulatory visits and the number of deaths. Non-Hispanic Black children have the lowest number of ambulatory visits and the highest number of deaths, but non-Hispanic White children have the highest number of ambulatory visits and the lowest number of deaths. This suggests a strong influence from social and environmental

Table 3-1

Asthma Prevalence, Health Care Use, and Mortality Among Children 0 to 17 Years of Age (By Race and Ethnicity United States, 2003 to 2005)

Race/ Ethnicity	Current Prevalence 2004 to 2005 (%)	Ambulatory Visits 2003 to 2004 (#/1000)	Emergency Department Visits 2003 to 2004 (#/10,000)	Hospital Discharges 2003 to 2004 (#/10,000)	Deaths 2003 to 2004 (#/1,000,000)
Hispanic	7.8	83.3	108.1	*	1.8
Puerto Rican	19.2	*	*	*	**
Mexican	6.4	*	*	*	1.7
Non-Hispanic White	8.0	100.2	65.8	*	1.3
Non-Hispanic Black	12.7	71.5	251.6	*	9.2
Asian	4.9	**	**	**	**
Total	**8.7**	**90.0**	**99.2**	**29.1**	**2.6**

*Data unavailable
**Data considered unreliable with relative standard error of the estimate greater than 30%

Adapted from Akinbami L. The state of childhood asthma, United States, 1980–2005. Advance data from *Vital and Health Statistics, Centers for Disease Control and Prevention.* 2006;381:1-28.

factors and indicates potential barriers to seeking appropriate outpatient care to establish asthma control rather than simply a genetic predisposition toward more brittle or severe asthma.

As the previously cited trends and statistics suggest, social, economic, racial, and gender-related factors are critical to asthma prevalence and severity. This is also reflected in the frequency and severity of what has been termed *inner-city asthma*. In the past several decades, it has become apparent that the burden of asthma has grown disproportionately among children residing in urban areas and particularly the inner cities of the United States. A multitude of factors are thought to contribute to this explosion of asthma among inner city children, many of whom are poor, socially and medically disadvantaged, and members of ethnic minority groups (Table 3-2). Factors such as poor living conditions, high levels of air pollution, the components of which can be immunomodifying and impact lung growth, and unique indoor allergens (eg, cockroach antigen) all contribute. Other factors, such as suboptimal access to medical care and inadequate care delivery, are important as well.

Table 3-2

Potential Contributory Factors in the Excess Burden of Asthma Among Children of Lower Socioeconomic Status

Health Care Systems Barriers	*Coexisting Medical Conditions*	*Psychosocial Challenges*	*Environmental Exposures*
Lack of access to care	Obesity	Low health literacy	Environmental tobacco smoke
Inadequacies of care	History of prematurity	Lack of education	Air pollution
Shortage of both primary and specialty physicians	Developmental or emotional problems	Lack of caregiver support	Cockroach antigen
Inability to afford medications		Family stress	Poor living conditions

Adapted from Jones CA, Clement LT. Inner city asthma. In: Leung DYM, Sampson HA, Geha RS, Szefler SJ. *Pediatric Allergy: Principles and Practice.* St. Louis, MO: Mosby; 2003.

Air pollution can have a major impact on children's respiratory health in many ways that are relevant to asthma. Air pollution is composed of many things, but particulate matter, nitrogen oxides, and ozone are most important to asthma and children's respiratory health. Levels of air pollution derived from the burning of fossil fuels can impact lung growth and function. Studies in Los Angeles have shown clear relationships between exposure to air pollution and levels of lung function in children. The closer a child lives to one of Los Angeles' famous freeways, the lower the level of his or her lung function. The individual components of air pollution can be toxic to the lung as well. Diesel exhaust particles have been shown to promote airway inflammation and modify the immune responses of airway epithelial cells, and truck traffic is an enormous contributor to toxic air pollution. Other components of smog, such as ozone, also cause lung inflammation.

Studies have shown clear relationships between levels of air pollution and asthma episodes in children. During the 1996 summer Olympic Games in Atlanta, the limitation of driving into the city during the games resulted in reduced air pollution that was clearly linked to reduced asthma morbidity in children. From these studies and others, it is clear that the quality of the air we breathe has important effects on children's respiratory health and asthma burden. While cause and effect are always very difficult to prove, perhaps it is not too surprising that asthma has begun to concentrate in urban areas that are sites of poor indoor, as well as outdoor, air quality. An important public health goal that has high relevance to asthma is to support legislation to minimize air pollution.

Currently in the United States, there is an asthma epidemic, with an unacceptably high prevalence of this disease among children during the past decades. This epidemic is not equally distributed, and the disproportionate burden of asthma borne by children residing in the inner cities and those of ethnic minority status is something that all clinicians should work to improve. Simply put, the differences in the impact of asthma vary by race, gender, and age. These differences place non-Hispanic Black teenage boys in the highest risk group of dying from asthma. They also emphasize the need to establish routine care in the ambulatory settings (especially in this group) because the number of ambulatory visits is inversely related to the number of deaths from asthma. Working to overcome barriers so that asthma care is equally accessible to all children is also an important goal. In the final analysis, all of us as pediatric providers will be treating a lot of children of all ages, races, and genders with asthma.

Suggested Readings

Akinbami L. The state of childhood asthma, United States, 1980–2005. Advance data from *Vital and Health Statistics, Centers for Disease Control and Prevention*. 2006;381:1-28.

Centers for Disease Control and Prevention. Vital signs: asthma prevalence, disease characteristics, and self-management education—United States 2001-2009. *MMWR*. 2011;60:1-7.

Friedman MS, Powell KE, Hutwagner L, Graham LM, Teague WG. Impact of changes in transportation and commuting behaviors during the 1996 Summer Olympic Games in Atlanta on air quality and childhood asthma. *JAMA*. 2001;285:897-905.

Gauderman WJ, Vora H, McConnell R, et al. Effect of exposure to traffic on lung development from 10 to 18 years of age: a cohort study. *Lancet*. 2007;369:571-577.

Jones CA, Clement LT. Inner city asthma. In: Leung DYM, Sampson HA, Geha RS, Szefler SJ. *Pediatric Allergy: Principles and Practice*. St. Louis, MO: Mosby; 2003.

The Asthma of Most of My Patients Seems Very Mild. Do Children Really Die From Asthma?

Robert A. Heinle, MD

Asthma is the most common chronic disease of childhood and is a condition often seen by pediatric health care providers. It is a condition that can be quite serious and even fatal. Thankfully, childhood deaths from asthma are rare, but they still do occur. Despite the fact that the majority of patients with asthma will never have a life-threatening episode, none of us should be lulled into a false sense of security because asthma is also a very variable condition that needs to be addressed thoroughly and with care. All patients need an individualized approach to their disease state, and a clear action plan for periods of wellness and periods of symptom exacerbation.

As with any health statistic, those regarding asthma death will be somewhat fluid and vary over time. With that caveat, in 2004, childhood deaths attributed to asthma occurred on the average of 2.5 deaths per 1 million children (186 children total). Besides the unimaginable human cost of this statistic, another additional disturbing aspect of asthma fatalities is the notion that asthma is a controllable disease with therapies that are both safe to prescribe and that have been shown to keep asthma patients protected from adverse outcomes, including death.

With early recognition, proper diagnosis of asthma and its comorbidities, initiation and monitoring of effective daily controller medications, and good adherence and technique of medication delivery by the patient and family, the number of asthma fatalities could be zero.

Deaths attributed to asthma had risen consistently during the 1980s and 1990s despite published diagnostic and therapeutic guidelines in 1991 (National Asthma Education and Prevention Program *Expert Panel Report*; NAEPP EPR). The cumulative mortality peaked in 1996 at 3.7 deaths per 1 million children. Subsequently, the mortality of asthma in children has been declining slowly but, as noted above, like any health statistic, asthma death rates will remain fluid.

Table 4-1
Important Risk Factors for Pediatric Asthma Death

- Asthma hospitalization in the previous 6 months
- Prior life-threatening asthma episode
- Medical deterioration in the previous month
- Recent use of oral corticosteroids
- Lack of adherence
- Short duration of final attack (<3 hours)
- Delay in seeking medical attention

Adapted from Jorgensen IM, Jensen VB, Vulow S, Dahm TL, Prahl P, Juel K. Asthma mortality in the Danish child population: risk factors and causes of asthma death. *Pediatr Pulmonol.* 2003;36:142-147.

Subgroup analysis shows that asthma mortality is not consistent across all demographics. Mortality due to asthma generally increases with age and male gender, with the highest mortality seen in boys ages 11 to 17 years, at a rate of 4.0 deaths per 1 million children in 2004. There is also disparity in mortality between racial ethnicities, with non-Hispanic Black children showing more than 7 times the mortality rate compared to non-Hispanic White children. In 2004, the mortality rate per 1 million was 1.3 deaths in non-Hispanic White children ages 0 to 17 years and 9.2 deaths in non-Hispanic Black children. This excessive burden in mortality is consistent with other data that show a higher incidence and severity of asthma in ethnic minorities and socially disadvantaged groups in the United States, even in 2011.

Consistent with published data about asthma mortality and the ongoing recognition of the variable and unpredictable nature of asthma, a change in philosophy occurred with the third expert panel report (NAEPP EPR-3). In this iteration of the guidelines, there was greater emphasis that disease severity (usually based on frequency of symptoms) does not predict the intensity of exacerbations and the specific recognition that dangerous exacerbations may occur with any severity of asthma, even intermittent asthma. This prompted the removal of the qualifier "mild" from the intermittent severity because even asthmatics with intermittent symptoms have the potential to have a severe life-threatening attack. This frame-shift was foreshadowed in the medical literature in the title of a retrospective study published in 1992 entitled "Pediatric Asthma Deaths in Victoria: The Mild Are at Risk."[1] An unforgettable message in this paper, that reviewed 51 asthma deaths during a 3-year period, was that 33% of the patients who died were considered by their physician to have had mild or even "trivial" asthma, and 32% of the patients who died had never been admitted to the hospital. Other important findings in this paper that have been noted repeatedly are the "importance of inadequate asthma assessment and therapy, poor compliance with therapy, and delay in seeking help" as risk factors for asthma death. A summary of the consistent risk factors for asthma death are noted in Tables 4-1 and 4-2.

Some other risk factors for a life-threatening asthma flare can be obtained from a patient's medical history. These include factors, such as previous severe exacerbations, that may have required admission to the pediatric intensive-care unit (PICU) or if a patient has ever required intubation for respiratory distress. Not surprisingly, previous

Table 4-2

Other Important Historical Factors to Consider in an Asthma Risk Assessment

- Asthma history
- Previous intensive-care unit admission
- Previous respiratory failure
- 2 or more asthma admissions or emergency department visits in the past year
- Hospitalization or emergency department visit for asthma in the previous month
- Using 2 or more canisters of short-acting beta-agonists per month
- Poor perception of asthma symptoms
- Atopy
- Lack of written asthma action plan
- Inner-city residence
- Low socioeconomic status
- Substance abuse
- Psychological comorbidity

intensive-care unit (ICU) admission and respiratory failure are associated with persistently increased asthma mortality. The lack of a written asthma action plan is a risk factor for poor outcome as are sensitivity to *Alternaria*, difficulty perceiving asthma symptoms, or the pattern of severity of exacerbations. Difficulty perceiving asthma symptoms has been associated with sudden and severe asthma attacks and is a particular concern because patients may not even realize how sick they are. Other factors may occur more remotely in the patient history, such as greater than one hospitalization or greater than 2 emergency department visits for asthma in the past year. More recent history may reflect risk factors, such as hospitalization or emergency department visit for asthma in the past month and using greater than 2 canisters of short-acting beta-agonists (SABA) per month.

The social history may also include risk factors for a life-threatening asthma exacerbation. Risk factors, such as inner city residence, low socioeconomic status, illicit drug use, or major psychosocial problems, all negatively impact the burden of asthma and result in increased risk of death. Finally, a patient may have comorbidities that are risk factors for increased mortality from asthma, including cardiovascular disease, other chronic lung disease, or chronic psychiatric disease.

These biological and psychosocial risk factors are so well characterized that it is easy to imagine a tool in the chart of all asthmatics in a pediatric practice or even emergency department that guides the practitioner through this important asthma risk assessment exercise when taking a patient history and developing an action plan for the patient. Assessing risk as an element of ongoing asthma management is completely in line with the latest asthma guidelines and is an important strategy to promote patient safety.

Appropriate asthma therapy is another means of promoting patient safety and helping to ensure a good clinical outcome. Inhaled corticosteroids are the first-line recommended controller therapy for persistent asthma. Not only do these agents safely and effectively treat the inflammation that underlies chronic asthma, inhaled corticosteroids have been demonstrated to prevent asthma fatalities as well. This unique characteristic of inhaled corticosteroids is further evidence to support their use as the drugs of choice for persistent asthma.

Though childhood deaths from asthma are rare, there are some patient characteristics and elements in a patient's history that may identify him or her as being at increased risk of dying from asthma. Similarly, the use of inhaled corticosteroids has been shown to reduce the risk of fatal asthma and should be the foundation of the care plan for any patient with persistent asthma, and particularly for those who are at increased risk of severe exacerbation or even asthma death. These epidemiological factors and medication interventions allow us to focus our efforts and motivate patients to increase the frequency and use of the ambulatory office visit to maintain asthma control and hopefully decrease the risk of death from asthma.

References

1. Robertson CF, Rubinfeld AR, Bowes G. Pediatric asthma deaths in Victoria: the mild are at risk. *Pediatr Pulmonol.* 1992;13:95-100.

Suggested Readings

Akinbami L. The state of childhood asthma, United States, 1980–2005. Advance data from *Vital and Health Statistics, Centers for Disease Control and Prevention.* 2006;381:1-28.

National Asthma Education and Prevention Program. *Expert panel report 3 (EPR-3): guidelines for the diagnosis and management of asthma.* Bethesda, MD: National Heart, Lung, and Blood Institute, 2007. NIH publication no. 08-4051.

Suissa S, Ernst P, Benayoun S, Baltzan M, Cai B. Low-dose inhaled steroids and the prevention of death from asthma. *N Engl J Med.* 2000;343:332-336.

Do Children Outgrow Asthma? What Is the Evolution of Asthma Throughout Childhood?

Robert A. Heinle, MD

Asthma and asthma-like episodes may actually encompass multiple etiologies in childhood. There is a broad differential diagnosis that must be considered when approaching a child with recurrent respiratory symptoms, especially at young ages when viral infections may cause bronchiolitis that mimics asthma. Other underlying medical or anatomic conditions may also be present. Similarly, asthma will evolve with the developing child, and this adds an additional layer of complexity to the management of childhood asthma. This is particularly the case when long-term controller therapy is being used to treat a condition that may eventually go into remission in an individual child.

Much has been learned from epidemiological studies about the evolution of asthma in childhood, including risk factors for its persistence and some of the complicating factors. For example, in children at risk for asthma, recurrent viral infections may allow a child to fulfill criteria for an asthma diagnosis for a period of time. Infants have such small airways that it may take very little inflammation or bronchoconstriction to induce wheezing. This is especially true in premature infants in whom there may be airway smooth muscle hyperplasia without significant inflammation, and their wheezing is often improved with bronchodilators. These are just a few of the confusing scenarios that are encompassed by the diagnosis of asthma that makes clarifying the natural history difficult.

Conducting controlled longitudinal studies to determine the natural history of asthma is also difficult. Changes in housing, family structure, and access to health care are difficult variables to control in our increasingly mobile society. In addition, variations in exposure to triggers, such as infections, air pollution, pets, environmental tobacco smoke, peer-group smoking, and occupational exposures, can also change over time and influence asthma symptoms and control. However, epidemiological studies are excellent sources of information about populations and trends, and the same is true for epidemiological studies about asthma. The challenge in clinical medicine is to translate these population-based data to the child in front of us in the office to determine the best possible plan of treatment. With these caveats, the following represents our current knowledge about the evolution of asthma throughout childhood.

Epidemiological studies of asthma have been performed in several westernized countries, including England, Australia, and the United States.[1-6] In the Tucson Children's Respiratory Study, a notable American study of the progression of childhood asthma, roughly 50% of all young children (younger than 3 years of age) in the study had "ever wheezed." Of this 50%, it was found that among 3-year-old children with a history of wheezing, 60% went on to "outgrow" their wheezing by 6 years of age. Termed *transient early wheezing*, infant pulmonary function testing was able to show that these children had decreased levels of pulmonary function early in life that persisted despite the resolution of their symptoms. As a group, they did not develop other asthma risk factors (see below). Therefore, this group of children likely had anatomic airflow obstruction due to small airways that contributed to their wheezing early in life. However, as they grew and as their lungs and airways grew, the resulting air flow was sufficient to enable them to become asymptomatic and demonstrate remission of airway symptoms.

The other 40% of children in the Tucson Children's Respiratory Study had persistent wheezing beyond the age of 6 years.[1] This translates to an approximately 20% rate of persistent wheezing in young children, a prevalence that has been found in epidemiologic studies from other westernized countries. Importantly, these children with persistent wheezing had significant risk factors for the development of asthma, airway inflammation, or worsened respiratory symptoms. These risk factors include eczema, rhinitis and wheezing apart from colds; elevated immunoglobulin-E (IgE) levels in the blood; a maternal history of asthma; a maternal history of smoking; frequent asthma symptoms during the first year of life; male gender; and Hispanic ethnicity. These risk factors are clinical parameters that can be explored at the bedside and help to quantify an individual patient's propensity to develop persistent asthma in childhood.

Similar results were seen in older children between 5 and 12 years of age where risk factors for asthma, such as allergen sensitization, exposure to indoor allergens, and increases in airway hyper-responsiveness, were all associated with more persistent airway symptoms. Additionally, decreased lung function, young age, and more severe asthma predicted persistence of symptoms that remained active in every quarter of the year (Table 5-1). Allergy testing, environmental history, and monitoring of symptoms are all important components of guideline-based asthma treatment that can also help with prognostication among pediatric patients.

The Childhood Asthma Management Program (CAMP) followed the lung function of children with mild to moderate asthma over a several-year period.[2] This study showed that asthma duration was strongly associated with decreased lung function, increased airway hyper-responsiveness, more asthma symptoms, and more frequent as-needed albuterol use. The children with more symptomatic asthma tended to have persistent symptoms.

Studies have estimated that between 40% and 60% of children with asthma will have resolution of their symptoms as adults. Longitudinal studies in the United States, England, and Australia suggest that the severity of asthma helps predict which children will have continued asthma symptoms. The majority (86%) of children at age 7 years with intermittent or mild asthma and few symptoms will continue to have little or no asthma as adults, whereas children with more frequent symptoms or severe asthma are more likely to continue to have asthma flares (71%). But, these studies also showed that nearly one third of the severe asthmatics had significant improvement in their symptoms as adults.

Table 5-1
Risk Factors for Persistence of Wheezing Into Adulthood

- Sensitization to house dust mites
- Airway hyper-responsiveness
- Female gender
- Smoking
- Early onset of symptoms
- Reduced lung function

Adapted from Sears MR, Greene JM, Willan AR, et al. A longitudinal, population-based cohort study of childhood asthma followed to adulthood. *N Engl J Med.* 2003;349:1414.

Summary

Wheezing and asthma-like symptoms are common throughout childhood, and a majority of children will have resolution of these episodes. Risk factors for asthma (atopy, elevated IgE, airway hyper-responsiveness, decreased lung function, and more severe asthma) may help identify children at risk for persistent asthma. As children with asthma enter adulthood, this resolution appears to continue for a majority of patients, but the children with more severe asthma during childhood are more likely to have persistence of symptoms in adulthood.

References

1. Martinez FD, Wright AL, Taussig LM, et al. Asthma and wheezing in the first six years of life. *N Engl J Med.* 1995;332:133.
2. Childhood Asthma Management Program Research Group. Long-term effects of budesonide or nedocromil in children with asthma. *N Engl J Med.* 2000;343:1054-1063.
3. Covar RA, Strunk R, Zeiger RS, et al. Predictors of remitting, periodic, and persistent childhood asthma. *J Allergy Clin Immunol.* 2010;125:359.
4. Morgan WJ, Stern DA, Sherrill DL, et al. Outcome of asthma and wheezing in the first 6 years of life: follow-up through adolescence. *Am J Resp Crit Care Med.* 2005;172:1253.
5. Zeiger RS, Dawson C, Weiss S. Relationships between duration of asthma and asthma severity among children in the Childhood Asthma Management Program. *J Allergy Clin Immunol.* 1999;103:376.
6. Sears MR, Greene JM, Willan AR, et al. A longitudinal, population-based cohort study of childhood asthma followed to adulthood. *N Engl J Med.* 2003;349:1414.

Suggested Readings

Weinberger M. Pediatric asthma and related allergic and nonallergic diseases: patient-oriented evidence-based essentials that matter. *Pediatric Health.* 2008;2:631.

SECTION II

ASTHMA PATHOPHYSIOLOGY

What Causes Asthma?
Is It Due to Genes, the Environment,
Infection, or Some Combination of These?

Katherine A. King, MD

In 1989, the cover of the journal *Science* had a picture of a child with a headline stating that the gene for cystic fibrosis had been isolated, and the medical future for people with this fatal genetic disease seemed much brighter.[1] Discussions among those of us at the pulmonary and allergy meetings in the 1990s focused on isolating the gene or genes responsible for asthma. The identification of these specific genes would provide clinicians with the ability to accurately diagnose this common disease, provide investigators with the means to understand the mechanisms of its pathophysiology, and give pharmaceutical companies the building blocks to make new and more effective therapies. Almost 20 years later, the current conclusion from all the promising research is that the causes of asthma are a combination of multiple genetic variations interacting with numerous environmental triggers, which may be further modulated by infectious diseases in early childhood.[2-4]

This revelation does not diminish the brightness of the new information about asthma genetics, nor the importance for clinicians to be aware of and actively involved in pursuing knowledge about asthma genes. In the 21st century, there are commercial diagnostic gene laboratories that analyze distinct genes, and this diagnostic methodology will be available when a consensus for an asthma gene panel has been achieved.[2]

The methodology for the analysis of asthma genes has taken 2 broad investigative approaches to address the important contributing parameters that induce the asthmatic response. Thus, investigators and clinicians need to work together to collect genotypic, phenotypic, and diagnostic clinical information from each patient cohort. One approach for the genetic analysis of a population is to collect a sample cohort of patients diagnosed with asthma, such as an ethnic population or a group of pediatric patients, and to compare the sample groups' genes with those from a control cohort of patients who do not have the clinical phenotype of asthma.[1,2] Then, using comparative genomic hybridization and positional cloning, the investigators attempt to determine if specific genes are mutated, up-regulated, or deficient in the asthma cohort. Last, these genes are then sequenced, and

---

Table 6-1

Examples of Candidate Asthma Genes and Their Putative Site of Action in the Airway and Pathogenetic Role

- Pulmonary capillary
  - PTGDR: Cell migration
- Airway smooth muscle
  - ADAM 33: Bronchial hyper-reactivity
  - Beta-adrenergic receptor polymorphisms: Bronchodilator response
- Lamina propria
  - Prostaglandin D synthase: Mast cell stimulation
- Airway epithelium
  - Toll-like receptor-2: Microbial pattern recognition

Adapted from Cookson W, Moffat M. Making sense of asthma genes. *N Engl J Med.* 2004;351:1794-1796.

---

the protein derived from the genetic sequence is isolated and then studied for its function within the lung. In this manner, the gene ADAM 33 coding for a bronchial smooth muscle protein was discovered in a selected asthmatic population.[2]

Another approach toward genetic analysis is to pick a pathway in the asthmatic cascade, such as the up-regulation of the immune response in asthmatic patients, and to study a candidate gene. Using a well-described asthma animal model, investigators hope to demonstrate that the candidate gene, which is either over-expressed or deficient in the animal model, will significantly disrupt the predictable asthmatic response in the animal model of interest. Then, these candidate genes can be targeted for study in a human asthmatic sample population. This was done for the PTGDR gene (prostaglandin D), which has an important role in T-cell chemotaxis.[2]

The analysis of one gene through bench science by a clinical investigator can provide the background knowledge for a pharmaceutical company to synthesize a drug to block or enhance the critical pathway. The dissemination and translation of this scientific knowledge to the public provides an additional challenge to us as clinicians. We must learn new genetic terms in order to address our families' questions about asthma genes and the genetic basis of this disease. This process is actively unfolding in the cystic fibrosis community today as the genetic discoveries of the past decades are translated into targeted cystic fibrosis genotype-based therapies.[1,2]

While asthma genetic research continues to narrow the search among the pathways that are the most important in the pathophysiology of asthma pathology, there are 10 genes already identified as asthma genes (Table 6-1). Selective proteins coded by these genes include structural proteins in the respiratory epithelium, airway proteases, chemotactic mediators, and enzymatic granules released by activated immune cells.[2] Thus, the current hypothesis suggests that while the asthma gene variations are present in the host, it is the exposure to environmental allergens and irritants and the infectious disease directives that propagate the asthmatic response of each patient over time.[3,4]

Table 6-2
Overview of TH1 and TH2 Cytokine Pathways

TH-1 Cytokine Pathway		TH-2 Cytokine Pathway	
Favors Cell-Mediated Immunity and Immunological Tolerance	**Activates**	**Favors Allergic Sensitization and Atopy**	**Activates**
Interleukin-2	B-cells	Interleukin-3	B-cells
Interleukin-3	Macrophages	Interleukin-4	Mast cells
Interferon-gamma	Natural killer cells	Interleukin-5	Eosinophils
	Cell-mediated immunity	Interleukin-6	
		Interleukin-9	
		Interleukin-13	

Multiple epidemiologic studies focusing on specific allergens and irritants demonstrate that the presence of dust-collecting clutter; high dust mite populations; environmental tobacco smoke exposure and smoking cigarettes; high pollen counts in humid summers; mold-infested homes, and homes along busy bus routes or highways that spew sulfides, nitrogen oxides, and particulate matter into the air significantly contributes to the genesis of asthma, induces asthma attacks, and impairs lung growth in pediatric patients.[3-5]

Prospective studies to analyze the effect of the environment on one mechanism of asthma, the induced immune response, are presented in the "Hygiene Hypothesis." The environmental differences of the 2 populations in western versus eastern Germany provide a natural laboratory to select comparative pediatric populations and demonstrate differences in atopy, infectious events, and asthma symptoms as well as environmental measurements of air pollution, bacterial endotoxins, dust presence, and sibling contagions. The breadth of the experimental setting shows a deviation of the developing immune response from that of one fighting over systemic and respiratory infections to one that releases mediators that cause mucosal thickening and airway bronchoconstriction, the cardinal features of asthma.[3]

The "Hygiene Hypothesis" states that, in the socially cleaner, upscale environment of western Germany, there are more asthma-like symptoms because the T-helper cell 2 (Th2) immune cells are producing allergy-promoting cytokines. In contrast, in the lower socioeconomic environment of eastern Germany, in which there are crowded family houses and farm animals in close proximity, the immune response remains skewed toward the T-helper cell 1 (Th1) response, which releases mediators that fight off infection and downregulate nonessential immune responses, such as seen in atopic individuals and those with asthma (Table 6-2).[3] These studies corroborate other American studies showing that children sent to daycare and those with many siblings tend to be sick as infants and young children but may be less likely to have asthma diagnosed at age 6 years.[4] These studies did not look at the potential asthma gene panel, but they did take into account family history and allergic sensitization and found these to be important, albeit imperfect, predictors of the presence of asthma at age 6 years. However, back home in our asthma clinics, we do tell our patients and their parents that while most children will grow out of wheezing and asthma symptoms by age 6 years, they should try to avoid triggering allergens and irritants in the environment. In addition, we can use tools such as the "asthma predictive index" to try and predict who will and will not "outgrow" their asthma symptoms.[5]

Infants and young children are exposed to viral and bacterial infections continuously. Up to 90% of all 2-year-olds have been exposed to the respiratory syncytial virus (RSV). Infections can decrease airway function on pediatric pulmonary function tests and potentiate asthma-like symptoms in young children.[5] This is particularly true of those with the genetic predisposition to atopy as measured by positive allergy tests. These infants and young children will most often develop recurrent respiratory symptoms consistent with asthma. The specific genes responsible for this predisposition, however, are not yet identified.[4,5]

It is clear that asthma, with its multiple pathophysiologic pathways and clinical phenotypes, results from a complex interplay of multiple genetic and environmental factors. The unavoidable viral and bacterial infections of childhood coupled with the genetic make-up of the individual child are critical. These are then further linked to critical environmental exposures to allergens or irritants. Together, this complex combination of stimuli and responses all combine to enhance respiratory symptoms and airway inflammation consistent with asthma. While the candidate genes that dominate these responses are being explored and will eventually be translated into specific therapies, those of us at the bedside are left with our clinical skills and intuition. We do not have a gene-based diagnostic kit, but the results of many large prospective epidemiological studies guide us in assessing risk and clinical parameters to assess the clinical severity. Thus, we all participate in a better understanding of childhood asthma.

References

1. Riordan JR, Rommens JM, Kerem B, et al. Identification of the cystic fibrosis gene: cloning and characterization of complementary DNA. *Science*. 1989;245:1066-1073.
2. Cookson W, Moffitt M. Making sense of asthma genes. *N Engl J Med*. 2004;351:1794-1796.
3. Braun-Fahrlander C, Riedler J, Hera U, et al. Environmental exposure to endotoxin and its relation to asthma in school-age children. *N Engl J Med*. 2002;347:869-877.
4. Martinez FD, Wright AL, Taussig LM, Holberg CJ, Halonen M, Morgan WJ; Group Medical Associates. Asthma in the first six years of life. *N Engl J Med*. 1995;332:133-138.
5. Castro-Rodriguez JA, Holberg CJ, Wright AL, Martinez ED. A clinical index to define risk of asthma in young children with recurrent wheezing. *Am J Respir Crit Care Med*. 2000;162:1403-1406.

WHAT IS THE ROLE OF AIRWAY INFLAMMATION IN ASTHMA?

Katherine A. King, MD

The classic definition of asthma, a condition characterized by reversible airway obstruction, has evolved into a complex medical disease. The understanding of the pathophysiology of asthma requires knowledge about genetic variations, the interaction between infectious agents and the respiratory epithelium, and the role of environmental allergens to modulate the patient's immune response.[1] Inflammation plays a central role in all of these factors. The specific role of inflammation in childhood asthma is the focus of several comprehensive prospective studies and is the basis of the National Institutes of Health's asthma care guidelines. In these studies, investigators strive to define the role of inflammation in asthma in order to provide better medical practice guidelines for clinicians taking care of patients with asthma.[1-4]

Clinicians are in the exciting position to evaluate young patients, who may be developing an asthma profile, and to participate in care plans to diminish the inflammatory process with both medical and lifestyle interventions. Three important clinical topics of discussion amidst the multitudes of clinical and basic science studies include: the innate and adaptive immune response, the reduction in measurable airway flow rates in the lower airways after respiratory infections in early childhood, and the observation that while inhaled steroids and immunotherapy do not cure or prevent asthma.[1,3,5,6]

Inflammation in the airway of a child with asthma is real and persistent. Chronic inflammatory cells have been isolated in the bronchial lavage fluid from the lower airways of children who have persistent wheezing.[1] Children with persistent wheezing are at risk of lower levels of lung function, and the chronic inflammation associated with asthma in childhood affects lung growth.[3]

Modern living standards and advances in medical care have not reduced the prevalence of asthma. An allergy-asthma coalition in Germany proposed the "Hygiene Hypothesis" after studying the impact of absorbing the population of eastern Germany into the German health care system.[6] The "Hygiene Hypothesis" proposes that, in the absence or reduction of microbial infections and bacterial endotoxins in the home environment, an allergic type of immune response is induced in a susceptible host. This immune response emphasizes the T-helper cell 2 (TH2) phenotype as opposed to the T-helper cell 1 (TH1) phenotype. The TH1 cytokine pathway results in cell-mediated immunity, which targets microbial infections, while the TH2 cytokine pathway favors the development of allergic inflammation. The predominance of TH2 activity leads to the release of pro-asthma cytokines and chemokines, such as interleukin 4 (IL-4), IL-5, and IL-13, which in turn mobilize and activate granular cells, such as eosinophils.[1,6] These eosinophils become activated and release arachidonic acid metabolites which lead to the synthesis of inflammatory mediators, such as prostaglandins and leukotrienes.[1,6] These activated cells and mediators then invoke the asthma symptoms of coughing, wheezing, and mucous hypersecretion. Medications, such as inhaled corticosteroids and leukotriene antagonists, target the cells and mediators that underlie these clinical phenomena.

The initiation and perpetuation of the inflammatory cascade begins with the stimulation of a TH2 cytokine response in a susceptible host. This cytokine response results in a downstream cascade that results in airway reactivity, epithelial extracellular edema, increased vascular permeability, and cellular mucous hypersecretion, which presents as the episodic wheezing and respiratory distress seen in persistent asthma and in asthma exacerbations.[1] The disruption of the regulation of a functional immune response, therefore, may present as an atopic child with difficult-to-control asthma. In medical practice, as clinicians, we will advocate avoidance of aero-allergens, such as dust mites or pollen, and the avoidance of irritants, such as tobacco smoke for children who have persistent wheezing because of the higher risk of exacerbations and the persistence of lower airway inflammation.[4]

As an interesting counterpoint, if the "Hygiene Hypothesis" is valid, we could advocate for the exposure to the right amounts of the right aero-allergens and infections at the right stage of development to switch the immune response toward the development of immunological tolerance and cell-mediated immunity (TH1 phenotype).[5] Theoretically, this switching of the immune response would decrease the risk of asthmatic inflammation. Obviously, this is not yet possible, and the risk of these types of recommendations currently outweighs any theoretical benefit. However, it provides a useful paradigm to consider when thinking about the roots of allergic inflammation.

The majority of children younger than 3 years of age have respiratory infections and will not have persistent wheezing. However, a prospective epidemiologic study called the Tucson Children's Respiratory Study demonstrated that a lower airway infection before the age of 3 years was a significant risk factor for persistent wheezing. This was shown by performing a specialized lung function test called the Maximal Expiratory Flow at Functional Residual Capacity (VMax-FRC).[3] Initially, at 1 year of age, there was no significant difference in the VMax-FRC between any of the pediatric patients with a history of wheezing. However, when the cohort of patients was retested at 6 years of age, those with a history of a significant wheezing-related lower airway respiratory tract infection before the age of 3 years had a significantly lower VMax-FRC as compared to those children who did not have a significant wheezing-related lower respiratory tract infection.[3]

This study is in agreement with members of the Australian and Canadian academic medical community who propose that nonallergic parameters in the lung, (eg, these viral lower respiratory tract infections) are also causative factors in asthma.[2,5] Their observations note that asthma-like respiratory symptoms are frequently documented in children with little evidence of atopy or exposure to passive smoking. The clinician's plan for appropriate medical therapy may begin with a discussion with the family to provide an understanding that recurrent wheezing in early childhood may be mediated by viral infections, and that specific interventions for allergies may not always be required. Good patient-physician communication is critical to bring home these points, and readily accessible medical care is important for the assessment of respiratory tract infections and the clinical management of persistent wheezing in children.

The importance of the role of inflammation in asthma is the crux of the National Heart Lung and Blood Institute of Health's asthma clinical practice guidelines in 2007.[4] This document includes evidence-based studies and a new approach to the guidelines that focuses on controlling asthma symptoms with an initial treatment plan, monitoring the patient's health, and then modifying the treatment plan as the asthma symptoms decrease. This approach reduces both the impairment and the risk from asthma symptoms and exacerbations, as well as from the adverse side effects of the medications. The guidelines advocate reduction of exposure to known allergens and irritating particulate matter. The guidelines recommend in children, even those younger than 5 years of age, the use of inhaled corticosteroids and leukotriene antagonists in order to decrease airway inflammation and to reduce the overuse of rescue medications.[4] This purposeful recommendation comes amidst ongoing concerns about medication side effects on the well-being, growth, organ development, and behavior of young children who have persistent childhood wheezing.

If chronic inflammation is the cause, then these medications might be expected to change the pathophysiology of asthma, but sadly, after weeks or months of inhaled steroid therapy in observed (clinical trial) settings, the respiratory symptoms return when the therapy stops.[3] Even other modes of treatment, such as immunotherapy, which are reported to restore the beneficial regulatory role of the T-cell to downregulate the immune response, or the injections of anti-immunoglobulin-E (IgE) antibodies do not redirect the misguided immune response or correct the structural changes in the lung. These anti-inflammatory therapies do restore quality of life and reduce the burden of asthma so that our patients are not sitting at home being sick, frequenting the emergency room, or being hospitalized for days.[1,5]

In the final analysis, a complex array of host genetic predispositions with environmental and infectious stimuli result in immunologic dysregulation that incites the asthmatic inflammatory cascade. Sometimes, this inflammation is clearly allergic, and, sometimes, it is primarily infection mediated.[2] This varying susceptibility is the basis for the broad array of symptoms which are experienced by patients with asthma. Inflammation is the reason for the proactive approach to start inhaled steroids in childhood to alter the immune response sufficiently to control persistent asthma and maintain positive immune response.

Summary

There is an important role of inflammation in childhood asthma. This scientific observation has substantiated the development of numerous anti-inflammatory medications, which are available to treat a patient with asthma. These medications have given both the clinician and the family the means to modulate the lung's immune response allowing the child to participate in an active lifestyle.

References

1. Leung DYM, Sampson HA, Geha RS, Szefler AJ, Eds. *Pediatric Allergy Principles and Practice*. St. Louis, MO: Mosby, Inc; 2003.
2. Kemp AS. Do allergens play a role in early childhood asthma? *Med J Aust*. 2002;177:S52-S54.
3. Martinez FD. Development of wheezing disorders and asthma in preschool children. *Pediatrics*. 2002;109: 362-367.
4. National Asthma Education and Prevention Program. *Expert panel report 3 (EPR-3): guidelines for the diagnosis and management of asthma*. Bethesda, MD: National Heart, Lung, and Blood Institute, 2007. NIH publication no. 08-4051.
5. McKay KO, Hogg JC. The contribution of airway structure to early childhood asthma. *Med J Aust*. 2002;177: S45-S47.
6. Braun-Fahrlander C, Riedler J, Herz U, et al. Environmental exposure to endotoxin and its relation to asthma in school-age children. *N Engl J. Med*. 2002;347:869-877.

WHAT IS THE DIFFERENTIAL DIAGNOSIS OF PEDIATRIC ASTHMA?

Natalie M. Hayes, DO and Aaron S. Chidekel, MD

Children with asthma often present with a variety of symptoms, but most commonly have cough, wheeze, or both. Because other diseases can also have such symptoms, it is important to consider if something other than asthma is going on or is contributing to the patient's symptoms. In many ways, the approach to a child with possible asthma is similar to the evaluation of a child with chronic or recurrent respiratory symptoms from any condition, and the possibilities, while not endless, are broad (Tables 8-1 and 8-2). With this in mind, it is best for the physician to develop a systematic approach to follow and guide the workup so that it may proceed selectively, yet efficiently, and decrease the likelihood that the diagnosis of a significant comorbidity or other condition will be delayed or overlooked completely.

Chronic cough is a common presenting complaint in pediatrics and is a frequent symptom of asthma. Cough is also a leading reason for a parent to seek medical evaluation for his or her child. It is a major economic factor in health care, and it can lead to unnecessary testing and treatment. It is, therefore, important that clinicians have familiarity with this common symptom when discussing its meaning with parents and patients, whether or not it results in the diagnosis of asthma being made. It is also critical that clinicians understand the pathophysiology of cough and its differential diagnosis so that treatment and investigations can be safe, efficient, and evidence based.

Cough is an important airway defense mechanism and is a vagally-mediated reflex with its afferent limb composed of mechano- and chemoreceptors throughout the oronasopharynx, larynx, and large and medium-sized airways. The efferent limb of the cough reflex is housed in the cough centers in the brainstem with cortical input as well. An intact cough reflex is critical to airway maintenance and clearance, and is a normal component of a functional respiratory system. In fact, healthy children may cough a little bit every day. The clinical evaluation of cough, therefore, should stem from the concept that cough is a symptom rather than a specific diagnosis, and, in many cases, the cough

Table 8-1

The Differential Diagnosis of Airway Abnormalities That May Mimic or Overlap With Pediatric Asthma

Upper Airway Disorders (Supraglottic and Glottic)	Large or Midsized Airway Obstruction (Tracheal and Bronchial)	Mid and Small Airway Obstruction (Bronchial and Bronchiolar)

• Allergic or nonallergic rhinitis
• Acute or chronic sinusitis
• Obstructive sleep apnea syndrome
• Exposure to irritants
• Vocal cord dysfunction
• Laryngomalacia
	• Airway foreign body
	• Airway anatomic abnormalities:
	  ○ Tracheomalacia
	  ○ Bronchomalacia
	  ○ Airway stenosis
	  ○ Vascular rings and slings
	  ○ Laryngeal web
	  ○ Subglottic cysts
	• Airway compression
	  ○ Cardiomegaly
	  ○ Benign thymic hyperplasia in infancy
	  ○ Lymph nodes
	  ○ Tumors
		• Viral bronchiolitis
		• Congestive heart failure
		• Bronchopulmonary dysplasia
		• Bronchiolitis obliterans
		• Suppurative lung disorders (see Table 8-2)

may be an expected or beneficial part of an illness or disease process. Other times, it may be a cause for significant concern.

The following characteristics can help to guide the evaluation and management of cough in childhood. On a temporal basis, cough can be considered acute, subacute (protracted), or chronic on the basis of the duration of the symptom. Most authorities agree that a chronic cough is a cough that has been present for longer than 4 weeks, while subacute and acute coughs have been present for 2 to 4 weeks and less than 2 weeks, respectively. The symptom of cough may be part of an identifiable underlying illness or syndrome, such as cystic fibrosis or immunodeficiency, or, far more commonly, the cough may be a manifestation of an intercurrent or acute problem, such as a viral respiratory tract infection. Rarely, cough may be due to a life-threatening situation, such as foreign-body aspiration. Finally, the specific quality of the cough may be recognizable or even diagnostic, such as those that occur with viral croup or pertussis (see Table 8-2). In general, features of cough that suggest asthma include a chronic dry and hacking cough that is worse at night, particularly in the middle of the night.

The evaluation of cough should be individualized based upon the patient history and physical examination. A critical component of the history is the environmental review, as exposure to environmental tobacco smoke is common and can, in and of itself, cause

Table 8-2

Common and Uncommon Cough Syndromes
That May Mimic or Overlap With Pediatric Asthma

Condition	Selected Clinical Clue
Asthma	Wheezing
Foreign body	Unequal breath sounds/wheezing
Pertussis	Paroxysmal coughing/inspiratory whoop
Chlamydia	Staccato cough/conjunctivitis
Croup	Barky cough/stridor
Tracheomalacia	Barky cough/stridor
Dysphagia/GER/aspiration	Cough may be associated with feeding
Suppurative lung disease*	Wet cough/clubbing/poor growth
Habit-Cough syndrome	Honking sound/absent during sleep
Unusual infections	Travel/environmental history
Hypersensitivity pneumonitis	Environmental history
Congenital airway abnormalities	Symptoms from birth
Unusual environmental exposures	Environmental history
Obsessive-compulsive disorder	Psychosocial history
Tourette's syndrome	Psychosocial history
Foreign body in the ear	Physical examination

*Examples of suppurative lung disorders include:
Protracted bacterial bronchitis
Cystic fibrosis
Noncystic fibrosis bronchiectasis
Right middle lobe syndrome
Primary ciliary dyskinesia
Immunodeficiency

chronic cough in childhood. Vaccination status and risk factors for exposure to infectious agents should also be noted as appropriate. In cases of acute or even protracted cough associated with a viral infection, no testing may be needed. Most authorities agree that, in cases of chronic cough, chest radiography should be obtained along with spirometry in children who can perform this maneuver. Other testing that may be recommended includes allergy testing, otorhinolaryngology evaluation, and sweat chloride analysis.

Similarly, the treatment of cough needs to focus on the underlying cause rather than the symptom of cough per se. Clinicians should remain sensitive to the concerns and needs of the patient and family but temper this with awareness of the relative ineffectiveness of cough suppressants and their potential dangers in selected populations, including the increased risk of adverse reactions in very young children and reported abuse of these

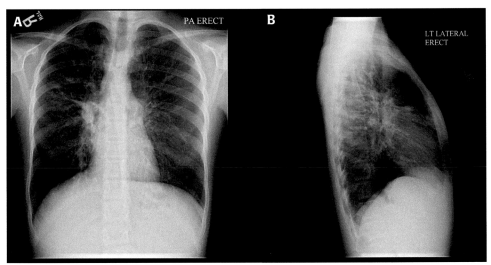

Figure 8-1. (A) Frontal and (B) lateral chest radiograph from an adolescent with mild to moderately severe cystic fibrosis. Hyperinflation and peribronchial thickening are seen and overlap with radiographic findings in asthma. Coarse interstitial markings and mucus plugging are more often seen in patients with cystic fibrosis, but also may be seen in asthma and other chronic airway diseases.

agents in adolescents. Therefore, in approaching a patient with the symptom of cough, the clinicians who adopt a thorough patient-centered approach rooted in the history and physical examination, and who understand and communicate the important aspects of this common clinical problem, will be able to evaluate children effectively, efficiently, and with sensitivity to the concerns of the family.

If the patient is acutely ill or is experiencing respiratory distress, consider the acute or potentially life-threatening conditions that will manifest with cough. Acute onset of symptoms would suggest a possible foreign-body aspiration, even if there was no known choking/gagging episode. If an aspiration occurred, chronic wheeze and cough that mimics asthma could develop. But, if either the patient or family members can pinpoint exactly when a symptom started, particularly if not associated with an upper respiratory tract illness, aspiration should be considered. Other causes of acute and severe cough include pertussis in a young infant, severe laryngotracheitis, bacterial tracheitis, or even severe asthma.

In approaching a subacute or chronic cough, the temporal and clinical characteristics will guide the differential diagnosis and evaluation. Viral infection will be the most common cause of acute coughing-related illnesses, while entities such as asthma and rhinosinusitis will predominate in cases of subacute and chronic cough. Allergy symptoms can cause postnasal drip, which can result in a cough. Patients with known atopy and/or signs or symptoms consistent with allergies such as shiners, Dennie lines, or a nasal crease/nasal salute sign will need appropriate treatment in order to alleviate symptoms. A chronic productive or moist cough suggests underlying suppurative lung disease such as cystic fibrosis or, more commonly, an entity known as protracted bacterial bronchitis in which the lower airway is colonized with pathogenic bacteria. Any child with a chronic cough and failure to thrive/falling off the growth curve should be evaluated for cystic fibrosis (Figure 8-1). Now that newborn screening (NBS) has been implemented in all

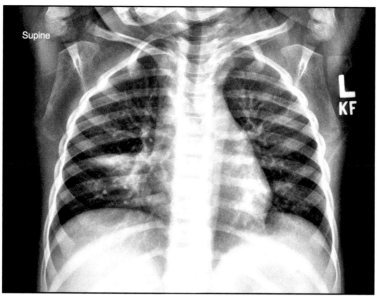

Figure 8-2. Typical chest radiograph from a patient with right middle lobe syndrome. In this patient, the right middle lobe is persistently collapsed, thereby increasing the risk of chronic infection and eventually the development of bronchiectasis. This patient has co-existing asthma complicated by recurrent lower respiratory tract infections. Flexible bronchoscopy did not reveal intrinsic or extrinsic obstruction of the right middle lobe bronchus, and bacterial cultures were negative.

50 states, hopefully, the majority of children with cystic fibrosis will be diagnosed in the newborn period. NBS is a screening tool, though, so it is still recommended to order a chloride sweat test for patients presenting in this way. Another example of a condition that results in a chronic, wet cough, while rare, is primary ciliary dyskinesia (PCD). Asthma and allergies might be the first thought given the persistent nasal drainage and cough that patients with PCD experience. However, frequent otitis media infections in addition to constant rhinorrhea raise the suspicion for PCD or immunodeficiency. Another red flag for PCD is a past medical history of respiratory distress soon after birth, such as transient tachypnea of the newborn. Other uncommon causes of chronic cough in childhood are non-CF bronchiectasis and right middle lobe syndrome (Figure 8-2). A more common example is gastroesophageal reflux (GER). Although the mechanisms and precise frequency of GER as a contributor to cough is controversial, GER is an important asthma co-morbidity. GER can present with cough, wheeze, or both, just like asthma. A cough at night soon after a child lies down or right after falling asleep is suspicious for reflux. Wheezing is a common finding in infants with reflux, and it may respond to a bronchodilator. However, complete relief is not sustained until reflux is treated.

In addition to cough, patients with asthma may present with chronic or recurrent episodes of wheezing or noisy breathing (Figures 8-3 and 8-4). It is helpful to consider noisy breathing as a manifestation of airway obstruction that may be due to asthma or another condition. An anatomic approach to noisy breathing (including wheezing) can be

Figure 8-3. Rigid bronchoscopic image of laryngomalacia obtained in an infant with chronic noisy breathing and retractions. The noisy breathing was primarily inspiratory and varied with activity in this patient.

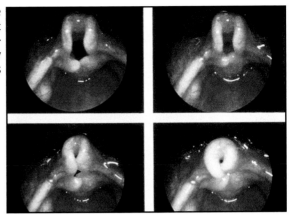

Figure 8-4. Rigid bronchoscopic image of a laryngeal web obtained in an infant with chronic noisy breathing and retractions. The noisy breathing was biphasic in this patient. Airway fluoroscopy was obtained as an initial screening study, and when found to be abnormal, the patient was referred for rigid bronchoscopy to allow for diagnosis and therapy of the airway lesion in one procedure. The web was resected with resolution of the patient's noisy breathing.

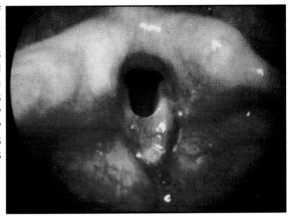

helpful in better defining the problem. In general, upper airway obstruction will result in inspiratory findings, while lower airway obstruction will result in expiratory findings. Central airway obstruction may result in inspiratory and expiratory findings. While this is a useful paradigm, practically, it may be difficult to distinguish stridor from wheezing and inspiratory findings from expiratory findings, particularly in a small child. In general, wheezing associated with asthma should be diffuse, expiratory, and responsive to bronchodilators. Characteristics other than this should alert the clinician to some of the other possible causes of noisy breathing in children. Although not common, one example of such a condition may be a vascular ring or sling. Imaging such as an upper gastrointestinal series or barium swallow may be able to determine if such an anatomic defect is present. Other examples of conditions associated with airway obstruction that are distinct from asthma were presented in Table 8-1. As with a child who has a chronic cough, the evaluation of a patient with chronic noisy breathing should proceed in a systematic fashion. Imaging studies and other more invasive testing such as bronchoscopy may be required to fully evaluate airway anatomy. Pulmonary function testing is helpful in quantifying airway obstruction but can be impractical in young children. If a true anatomic abnormality is detected, the treatment will be specific to the lesion.

Summary

The differential diagnosis of pediatric asthma is broad but not infinite. While asthma is the most common chronic respiratory condition affecting children, there is significant overlap between the presentation of asthma and other potentially serious pediatric respiratory disorders. Therefore, a thorough but sensible evaluation is important. Additionally, because the symptoms of asthma, namely coughing, wheezing, and increased work of breathing, are also nonspecific, a thorough understanding of the other entities in pediatrics that also present with these features is necessary. Familiarity with airway anatomy and physiology is also critical to allow for targeted testing. By evaluating each patient individually with this differential diagnosis in mind, it is unlikely that a serious condition that overlaps with asthma will be overlooked.

Suggested Readings

Carr BC. Efficacy, abuse, and toxicity of over-the-counter cough and cold medicines in the pediatric population. *Curr Opin Pediatr.* 2006;18:184-188.

Chang AB, Landau LI, Van Asperen PP, et al. Cough in children: definitions and clinical evaluation. *Med J Aust.* 2006;184:398-403.

Chang AB, Lasserson TJ, Gaffney J, Connor FL, Garske LA. Gastro-oesophageal reflux treatment for prolonged non-specific cough in children and adults. *Cochrane Database Syst Rev.* 2006;4:CD004823.

Chipps BE. The evaluation of infants and children with refractory lower respiratory tract symptoms. *Ann Allergy Asthma Immunol.* 2010;104:279-283.

Hayes NM, Chidekel A. Pediatric choking. *Del Med J.* 2004;76:335-340.

Kemp A. Does post-nasal drip cause cough in childhood? *Paediatr Respir Rev.* 2006;7:31-35.

National Asthma Education and Prevention Program. *Expert panel report 3 (EPR-3): guidelines for the diagnosis and management of asthma.* Bethesda, MD: National Heart, Lung, and Blood Institute, 2007. NIH publication no. 08-4051.

Weinberger M, Abu-Hasan M. Pseudo-asthma: when cough, wheezing, and dyspnea are not asthma. *Pediatrics.* 2007;120:855-864.

Weiss LN. The diagnosis of wheezing in children. *Am Fam Physician.* 2008;77:1109-1114.

How Do I Know It Is Asthma That Is Causing My Patient's Symptoms?

Anita Bhandari, MD

Asthma is the most common chronic disease in childhood, affecting about 12.7% of American children. In 2005, 9 million children were diagnosed with asthma at some point in their lifetime, 70% of which were reported to have a current diagnosis of asthma. Almost two thirds of these children were said to have at least one asthma exacerbation in the preceding 12 months. Pediatric asthma is associated with considerable morbidity. United States National Health Interview Survey data from 2003 reveal that asthma accounts for approximately 12.8 million missed school days. In 2003, there were 750,000 visits to emergency departments for asthma and 198,000 hospitalizations for asthma; in 2004, 7 million ambulatory visits were made for asthma.[1]

Asthma is defined as a chronic inflammatory disease of the airways. This airway inflammation causes several things that lead to acute airway obstruction, including an increase in bronchial hyper-responsiveness, airway edema, and mucous production (Table 9-1). Each of these contributes to recurrent episodes of wheezing, breathlessness, chest tightness, and coughing. These symptoms are usually associated with widespread but variable airflow obstruction, which is often reversible. These factors should respond to a trial of medications that can be used clinically to help tease out the diagnosis. Longstanding airway inflammation can result in airway smooth muscle hypertrophy and collagen deposition that is less reversible or possibly even irreversible as a process called airway remodeling evolves (see Table 9-1). This inflammation-based definition provides a basis for both diagnosis and treatment of asthma, as well as providing a strong clinical rationale for providing anti-inflammatory therapies.

Making a diagnosis of asthma in children can be challenging, especially in infants and young children. There are no diagnostic tests for asthma for infants and preschoolers, and a tentative diagnosis is usually made solely on the basis of clinical history and exam. Symptoms are usually recurrent, usually occur in response to a trigger, and are responsive to asthma therapy—the 3 Rs of asthma.

Table 9-1

Major Mechanisms of Airway Obstruction in Asthma

Reversible	*Less Reversible (Airway Remodeling)*
• Bronchoconstriction • Airway edema • Mucous hypersecretion/plugging • Epithelial sloughing	• Airway smooth muscle hypertrophy • Epithelial basement membrane thickening

Common symptoms of asthma include recurrent wheezing, chronic cough that is typically worse at night, recurrent episodes of difficulty breathing, chest tightness, and sputum production. Symptoms may be perennial or seasonal; there may be diurnal variations such that they may be more prominent upon first awakening in the morning or may be only nocturnal. These symptoms should be relieved when a patient is treated with asthma therapy, including inhaled bronchodilators and inhaled or oral steroids. There may be many precipitating factors, such as viral upper respiratory tract infections, exercise, and exposures including mold, dust mites, cockroaches, animal dander, pollen, cold air, and tobacco smoke. Emotions and stress can also be a trigger in some patients. Obtaining environmental history is important and may shed light on an otherwise unrecognized precipitating factor. Because there is a strong genetic predilection to asthma and other atopic diseases, a positive family history of asthma and/or atopy makes the diagnosis of asthma more likely.

During an acute episode, patients may have signs of increased work of breathing such as higher respiratory rates, nasal flaring, and intercostal and subcostal retractions. On auscultation, they may have decreased air entry or diffuse heterophonous wheezing and a prolonged expiratory phase and decreased oxygen saturation on pulse oximetry. These signs and symptoms improve with bronchodilator therapy, a test that can easily be done in the primary care provider's office. In between acute episodes, patients often have a completely normal chest exam. Most school-aged children with asthma have allergies, so stigmata such as allergic shiners, nasal allergic creases, and atopic dermatitis may be present if the patient has a significant history of atopy. Presence of allergic stigmata supports the diagnosis of asthma. Presence of clinical findings such as digital clubbing, failure to thrive, absence of tonsillar tissue, hepatosplenomegaly, lymphadenopathy, and presence of heart murmurs are unusual with asthma and suggest alternative diagnoses.

In toddlers with a history of four or more episodes of wheezing with at least one physician diagnosis or history of four or more episodes of wheezing with at least one confirmed by a physician, Taussig and colleagues[2] described an asthma predictive index that is a statistically optimized algorithm to identify toddlers with wheezing who are likely to develop persistent asthma. A positive asthma predictive index includes recurrent episodes of wheezing in the past 1 to 2 years as well as one of the 2 major criteria or 2 minor criteria. Major criteria include physician-diagnosed atopic dermatitis or physician-diagnosed parental asthma. Minor criteria include physician-diagnosed allergic rhinitis, wheezing

Table 9-2
Modified Asthma Predictive Score

Major Criteria	*Minor Criteria*
Parental history of asthma	Allergic sensitization to milk and peanuts
Physician-diagnosed atopic dermatitis	Wheezing unrelated to colds
Allergic sensitization to at least 1 aero-allergen	Blood eosinophils ≥4%

Child must have a history of 4 or more episodes of wheezing with at least 1 episode confirmed by a physician.

Adapted from Guilbert TW, Morgan WJ, Zeiger RS, et al. Atopic characteristics of children with recurrent wheezing at high risk for development of childhood asthma. *J Allergy Clin Imunol.* 2004;114:1282-1287.

apart from colds, and peripheral blood eosinophilia. They reported that, in their study cohort, 68% of children with negative asthma predictive index never developed symptoms suggestive of asthma during their school years. In contrast, three-fourths of the children with a positive asthma predictive index developed symptoms of active asthma at least once. Guilbert and colleagues[3] have proposed a modified index (Table 9-2) in which they have included symptoms of atopy as well. They postulated that infants and preschoolers with wheezing who meet these criteria are at a higher risk of developing persistent asthma and that this risk may be related to early allergic sensitization. Simple, clinically based criteria such as these may be used to counsel families and accurately predict the outcome of disease in some patients.

In patients older than 5 years of age, spirometry may be attempted. On spirometry, presence of obstructive lung disease as suggested by a low FEV1, decreased FEV1/FVC ratio, and normal FVC supports the diagnosis of asthma. Furthermore, improvement in FEV1 by 10% to 12% following bronchodilator therapy, which is called a "positive bronchodilator response," is also considered supportive of a diagnosis of asthma. Methacholine challenge and exercise challenge are bronchoprovocation tests that may also be obtained to confirm airway hyper-reactivity. Often, patients with mild asthma may have no abnormality on spirometry, whereas those with severe or inadequately treated asthma may. Chest x-ray can also be obtained, but chest x-ray findings are nonspecific and may include hyperinflation, atelectasis, or signs of airway inflammation, such as peribronchial thickening. Elevated nitric oxide concentration in the exhaled air suggests airway inflammation and is considered supportive of a diagnosis and is used to distinguish asthma from other causes of chronic cough. Induced sputum for presence of eosinophils has limited use in children.

It is important to remember that "all that wheezes is not asthma." Some clues that suggest an alternative diagnosis are presence of symptoms since birth, presence of stridor, cough and wheeze associated with feeding, sudden onset of cough and wheeze, failure to thrive, history suggestive of malabsorption, or a persistent wet or juicy cough. If your patient is not responding to usual asthma medications, other differential diagnostic entities as shown in Table 9-3, for example, cystic fibrosis, tracheomalacia (Figure 9-1), gastroesophageal reflux, recurrent sinusitis, underlying immunodeficiency, and ciliary

Table 9-3

Other Causes of Coughing and Wheezing in Childhood

Infants	Preschoolers	School Age
GER	Cystic fibrosis	Cystic fibrosis
Cystic fibrosis	Ciliary dyskinesia	Ciliary dyskinesia
Congenital abnormalities of lung and airways (vascular rings/sling, tracheomalacia, bronchomalacia)	Foreign body inhalation	Immunodeficiency
Ciliary dyskinesia	Aspiration	alpha-1 antitrypsin deficiency
Congenital heart disease	Immunodeficiency	Vocal cord dysfunction
Immunodeficiency	Right middle lobe syndrome	Malignancies
Bronchopulmonary dysplasia	Protracted bacterial bronchitis	
Right middle lobe syndrome		

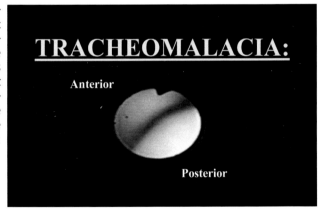

Figure 9-1. This is a flexible bronchoscopic image from an infant with noisy breathing caused by tracheomalacia. The airway should be a semi-rigid and patent tube. This image demonstrates the dynamic airway collapse associated with tracheomalacia as indicated by the anterior and posterior wall of the airway coming together, resulting in variable airway obstruction.

dyskinesia (Figure 9-2), need to be considered. Presence of restrictive lung disease, absence of bronchodilator response on spirometry, or presence of persistently abnormal radiographic findings should also prompt consideration of an alternative diagnosis. Causes of recurrent cough and wheeze may vary with the age of the child, and a broad differential as shown in Table 9-3 needs to be considered.

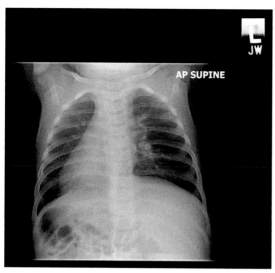

Figure 9-2. Chest radiograph obtained in an infant with classic ciliary dyskinesia with situs inversus (Kartagener syndrome). Note the dextrocardia and right-sided stomach bubble. Ciliary dyskinesia is a rare disorder associated with recurrent sino-pulmonary infections that is often accompanied by a severe asthma syndrome with chronic cough and wheeze. Unfortunately, it is rarely this obvious, and ciliary function disorders can be difficult to confirm.

References

1. Akinbami LJ. The state of childhood asthma, United States,1980-2005. *Adv Data*. 2006;381:1-24.
2. Taussig LM, Wright AL, Holberg CJ, Halonen M, Morgan WJ, Martinez FD. Tucson children's respiratory study 1980 to present. *J Allergy Clin Imunol*. 2003;111:661-675.
3. Guilbert TW, Morgan WJ, Zeiger RS, et al. Atopic characteristics of children with recurrent wheezing at high risk for development of childhood asthma. *J Allergy Clin Imunol*. 2004;114:1282-1287.

SECTION III

ASTHMA THERAPY

WHAT ARE THE COMMON CLASSES OF ASTHMA MEDICATION AND HOW DO THEY WORK?

Lisa Forbes, MD and Jonathan M. Spergel, MD, PhD

Because pharmacologic intervention is the mainstay of treatment for asthma, it is important to think of initiating treatment in a stepwise fashion. The 2007 National Asthma Education and Prevention Program (NAEPP) is based on increasing medications until asthma is controlled and, in turn, decreasing them to minimize potential side effects when possible. Table 10-1 lists the current categories of asthma medications used to treat acute exacerbations, as well as those used for daily therapy. Resources are available online that provide up-to-date branded information about currently available inhaled asthma medications. One example of a poster that can be purchased can be found at the Web site of the Allergy & Asthma Network Mothers of Asthmatics (www.breatherville.org or www.aanma.org).

Controller Medications

INHALED CORTICOSTEROIDS

Inhaled corticosteroids (ICS) are now the preferred controller therapy for persistent asthma based on current US and world guidelines (Table 10-2). They come in 3 forms: nebulized (budesonide [Pulmicort Respules; AstraZeneca, Wilmington, Delaware]), dry powder inhalers (mometasone furoate [Asmanex Twisthaler; Merck & Co. Inc, Kenilworth, New Jersey] or budesonide [Pulmicort Flexhaler; AstraZeneca]), and metered-dose inhalers (MDI; beclomethasone [QVAR; Teva Pharmaceuticals Industries Ltd, Petah Tikva, Israel], fluticasone [Flovent; GlaxoSmithKline, Brentford, Middlesex, United Kingdom], triamcinolone [Azmacort; Abbott Laboratories, Kennett Square, Pennsylvania], ciclesonide [Alvesco; Sunovion, Malborough, Massachusetts], or flunisolide [Aerobid; Forest

---

Table 10-1

Asthma Medications

Reliever medications:	Controller medications:
• Short-acting β_2 agonists • Anticholinergic bronchodilators • Short-term oral corticosteroids	• Inhaled corticosteroids • Long-acting β_2 agonists (monotherapy NOT recommended) • Leukotriene modifiers • Nonsteroidal anti-inflammatory agents • Methylxanthines • Anti-immunoglobulin-E monoclonal antibody therapy • Daily oral corticosteroids

---

Table 10-2

Inhaled Corticosteroid Fun Facts From the *Expert Panel Report 3*

- Inhaled corticosteroids are the preferred agents for treating persistent asthma
- Inhaled corticosteroids are the most potent and efficacious controller medications
- Inhaled corticosteroids are used daily and long-term to control asthma
- Inhaled corticosteroids benefits are most notable at low to medium doses
- Inhaled corticosteroids come in metered-dose inhaler, dry powder inhaler, or aerosol solution forms
- Inhaled corticosteroids are safe to use, even in young children
- Inhaled corticosteroids decrease airway inflammation and hyper-responsiveness
- Inhaled corticosteroids improve lung function

Adapted from National Asthma Education and Prevention Program. *Expert panel report 3: guidelines for the diagnosis and management of asthma.* Bethesda, MD: National Heart, Lung, and Blood Institute, 2007. NIH publication no. 08-4051.

Laboratories Inc, New York, New York]). These medications act through the glucocorticoid receptors (GRs) in the cytoplasm. The steroid molecules differ in their binding affinities to the glucocorticoid receptor, their metabolism in the hepatic tract, and their distribution in the body. When the molecules enter the cell, they then bind to the GR. The receptors undergo structural changes, disassociate the carrier proteins, and expose the nuclear localization signals to the GR. The corticosteroid (CS)/GR complex quickly translocates to the nucleus of the cell and binds to specific DNA sequences in gene promoter regions. The CS can promote or inhibit gene expression. It promotes anti-inflammatory gene production such as IL-10, beta-2 adrenergic receptor gene, and NF-κB inhibitor gene. Similarly, it inhibits pro-inflammatory gene production by inhibiting the NF-κB and AP-1 pathways, among others.

After inhaling CS, approximately 10% to 20% of the dose delivered is deposited in the lungs as most of the medication impacts on the oropharynx and is swallowed. Three systematic reviews show that budesonide, fluticasone, and beclomethasone promote improvement in forced expiratory volume in the first second (FEV1) and peak expiratory flow rate (PEFR). They have been shown to lower the frequency of asthma exacerbations, improve asthma symptoms, and decrease the need for beta-2 agonists when given in any daily dose versus placebo. The Prevention of Early Asthma in Kids (PEAK) trial found that ICS provided benefit in terms of episode-free days, emergency department visits, hospitalizations in the past year, and daily symptoms at baseline. Children with allergen sensitization had better control and had less oral corticosteroid use, fewer urgent care visits, and less use of supplemental controller medications. It has also been suggested that the use of high-dose ICS in preschool-age children reduced the use of rescue oral CS.

ICS use in children is also safe. The effect on height has been only seen in the first year of use, and in long-term follow-up, patients reach normal adult height.[1-3] There have been very rare reported cases of suppression of the hypothalamic-pituitary axis. Patients treated with low to moderate doses of ICS usually do not have significant changes in 24-hour plasma cortisol levels in response to adrenocorticotropic hormone (ACTH) stimulation. There is little significant change in bone markers or degradation in children treated with ICS.[4-8] Overall, the many benefits from ICS far outweigh any risks, and ICS are the recommend controller medications for asthma.

LEUKOTRIENE BLOCKERS

The leukotriene receptor antagonists (montelukast [Singulair] or zafirlukast [Accolate]) and 5-lipoxygenase inhibitors (zileuton [Zyflo]) were developed to treat the pro-inflammatory mediators released during asthma-related inflammation not treated by CS. Cystienyl leukotrienes cause bronchoconstriction, mucous secretion, and increased vascular permeability, and they promote smooth muscle proliferation and eosinophil migration to the airways. Montelukast, one of the receptor blockers, has also been shown to attenuate exercise-induced bronchospasm.[9-12] In one study, it produced improvements in daytime and nighttime symptom scores, days with asthma symptoms, and the need for beta-2 agonists or oral steroid, and it demonstrated this effect regardless of ICS use in patients 2 to 5 years of age. It was also shown to attenuate asthma exacerbations in children.[13]

Montelukast has a positive safety profile, and the most commonly reported adverse reactions were upper respiratory infection, worsening asthma, and fever for all treatments in the study including placebo.[14] There are reports about changes in behavior with montelukast. However, there are insufficient data to prove there is a link between montelukast and suicidality.[15]

LONG-ACTING BRONCHODILATORS

There are two long-acting bronchodilators that are currently available (salmeterol [Serevent] and formoterol [Foradil]). These beta-2 agonists have the same mechanism of action as short-acting beta-2 adrenergic receptor agonists, except they exert their effect for 12 hours. In addition, they also inhibit mast cell mediator release and plasma exudation, and they may reduce sensory nerve activation. Randomized controlled studies have shown that adding a long-acting bronchodilator to an ICS improves symptom control and lung function and reduces asthma exacerbations when compared to higher doses of ICS alone.[16-18] Clinical studies have demonstrated that the long-acting bronchodilators plus ICS is superior to either ICS or long-acting bronchodilators alone.

These medications are never to be used as a single agent in treating asthma and are only used in conjunction with other controller medications, primarily ICS (Advair [fluticasone-salmeterol], Symbicort [budesonide-formoterol], Dulera [mometasone/formoterol]). The long-acting bronchodilators have a black warning when used as a single agent; however, there is controversy about whether the warning should remain if a long-acting bronchodilator is included with an ICS[19] (the Food and Drug Administration currently has the warning).

Phosphodiesterase Inhibitors (Theophylline)

Theophylline is inexpensive and widely available. It is reserved as a third-line treatment for difficult-to-control asthma. It exerts its anti-inflammatory effects through phosphodiesterase inhibition, adenosine receptor antagonism, increase in IL-10 release, inhibition of NF-κB nuclear translocation, and the activation of histone deacetylase. It also enhances the anti-inflammatory effects of CS. There is increasing evidence that, at lower doses, it has an anti-inflammatory effect and can be an effective adjuvant therapy to patients with severe asthma. The side effects include nausea, vomiting, and headaches. Cardiac arrhythmias and seizures are possible but are rarely seen at plasma concentrations less than 10 mg/L.[20-26] Due to these side effects and the need to follow serum levels, along with the availability of more efficacious ICS agents, the use of theophylline and related agents has decreased markedly in recent years.

Mast Cell Stabilizer

There are two mast cell stabilizers (cromolyn and nedocromil [Tilade]). They are best used as adjuvant therapy for patients not well controlled on inhaled steroids alone. As an effective steroid-sparing addition to asthma therapy, both mast cell stabilizers show added benefit in reduction of symptoms without any loss of effect of inhaled steroids. These medications are safe and easy to use, but, as with the phosphodiesterase inhibitors, their use has also dropped off in recent years.[27] Mast cell stabilizers are further discussed in Question 12.

Reliever Medications

There are 2 basic outpatient reliever medications: bronchodilators and systemic anti-inflammatory medications.

Short-Acting Selective Beta-2 Agonists

The beta-2 adrenoreceptor gene is expressed on bronchial smooth muscle cells, and activation of these receptors induces smooth muscle dilation in response to endogenous catecholamines or exogenous triggers. Albuterol, a short-acting bronchodilator (SABA), acts on these receptors during an acute exacerbation to dilate smooth muscle. Its onset of action is short with effective bronchodilation achieved within 15 minutes of inhalation. The duration of action is 4 to 6 hours. Albuterol comes in several forms (oral, inhaled via

Table 10-3
Long Term Side Effects of Oral Corticosteroids

- Osteopenia
- Osteoporosis
- HPA-axis suppression
- Hypertension
- Cushingoid features
  - Moon facies
  - Central obesity
  - Striae
- Glucose intolerance
- Diabetes
- Skin thinning and easy bruising

nebulizer, or MDI). Inhaled versions have significantly fewer side effects as compared to the oral formulation. The nebulizer dose is equivalent to MDI in terms of efficacy. Both the MDI and nebulized forms come as either racemic or single isomer form (levalbuterol [Xopenex]). The side effect profiles of racemic and single isomer albuterol are equivalent at dose levels. In some studies, levalbuterol was as effective as racemic albuterol at half the dose; however, this finding has not been reproduced in other studies. SABA is the treatment of choice for acute asthma exacerbation management. This class of medication is well-tolerated by pediatric patients. Common side effects include tachycardia, nausea, nervousness, and decreased serum potassium.[28]

ORAL GLUCOCORTICOIDS

With the onset of ICS therapy, oral corticosteroid use is reserved for acute asthma exacerbations or for severe patients who cannot be controlled on ICS with long-acting bronchodilators alone. The mechanism of action of oral glucocorticoids is the same as ICS; however, the systemic absorption is greater. Although, the anti-inflammatory response is greater with oral therapy, it comes with more side effects (Table 10-3). Long-term use can leave the patient susceptible to growth delay, osteopetrosis and osteoporosis, abnormal glucose metabolism, and hypertension. In the short term, the patient can experience irritability, difficulty with sleep, and increase in appetite.

References

1. Barnes PJ. Anti-inflammatory actions of glucocorticoids: molecular mechanisms. *Clin Sci (Lond)*. 1998;94: 557-572.
2. Barnes NC, Hallett C, Harris TA. Clinical experience with fluticasone propionate in asthma: a meta-analysis of efficacy and systemic activity compared with budesonide and beclomethasone dipropionate at half the microgram dose or less. *Respir Med*. 1998;92:95-104.
3. Adams NP, Jones PW. The dose-response characteristics of inhaled corticosteroids when used to treat asthma: an overview of Cochrane systematic reviews. *Respir Med*. 2006;100:1297-1306.

4. Hopp RJ, Degan JA, Phelan J, Lappe J, Gallagher GC. Cross-sectional study of bone density in asthmatic children. *Pediatr Pulmonol.* 1995;20:189-192.
5. Allen DB. Safety of inhaled corticosteroids in children. *Pediatr Pulmonol.* 2002;33:208-220.
6. Bacharier LB, Guilbert TW, Zeiger RS, et al. Patient characteristics associated with improved outcomes with use of an inhaled corticosteroid in preschool children at risk for asthma. *J Allergy Clin Immunol.* 2009;123:1077-1082, 82 e1-5.
7. Harding SM. The human pharmacology of fluticasone propionate. *Respir Med.* 1990;(84 Suppl A):25-29.
8. Bush A. Practice imperfect—treatment for wheezing in preschoolers. *N Engl J Med.* 2009;360:409-410.
9. Busse WW. The role of leukotrienes in asthma and allergic rhinitis. *Clin Exp Allergy.* 1996;26:868-879.
10. Laitinen LA, Laitinen A, Haahtela T, Vilkka V, Spur BW, Lee TH. Leukotriene E4 and granulocytic infiltration into asthmatic airways. *Lancet.* 1993;341:989-990.
11. Drazen JM, Israel E, O'Byrne PM. Treatment of asthma with drugs modifying the leukotriene pathway. *N Engl J Med.* 1999;340:197-206.
12. Leff JA, Busse WW, Pearlman D, et al. Montelukast, a leukotriene-receptor antagonist, for the treatment of mild asthma and exercise-induced bronchoconstriction. *N Engl J Med.* 1998;339:147-152.
13. Johnston NW, Mandhane PJ, Dai J, et al. Attenuation of the September epidemic of asthma exacerbations in children: a randomized, controlled trial of montelukast added to usual therapy. *Pediatrics.* 2007;120:e702-e712.
14. Bisgaard H, Skoner D, Boza ML, et al. Safety and tolerability of montelukast in placebo-controlled pediatric studies and their open-label extensions. *Pediatr Pulmonol.* 2009;44:568-579.
15. Manalai P, Woo JM, Postolache TT. Suicidality and montelukast. *Expert Opin Drug Saf.* 2009;8:273-282.
16. Pauwels RA, Lofdahl CG, Postma DS, et al. Effect of inhaled formoterol and budesonide on exacerbations of asthma. Formoterol and Corticosteroids Establishing Therapy (FACET) International Study Group. *N Engl J Med.* 1997;337:1405-1411.
17. Bateman ED, Hurd SS, Barnes PJ, et al. Global strategy for asthma management and prevention: GINA executive summary. *Eur Respir J.* 2008;31:143-178.
18. Greening AP, Ind PW, Northfield M, Shaw G. Added salmeterol versus higher-dose corticosteroid in asthma patients with symptoms on existing inhaled corticosteroid. Allen & Hanburys Limited UK Study Group. *Lancet.* 1994;344:219-224.
19. Taylor DR. The beta-agonist saga and its clinical relevance: on and on it goes. *Am J Respir Crit Care Med.* 2009;179:976-978.
20. Dent G, Giembycz MA, Rabe KF, Wolf B, Barnes PJ, Magnussen H. Theophylline suppresses human alveolar macrophage respiratory burst through phosphodiesterase inhibition. *Am J Respir Cell Mol Biol.* 1994;10:565-572.
21. Persson CG. Development of safer xanthine drugs for treatment of obstructive airways disease. *J Allergy Clin Immunol.* 1986;78(4 Pt 2):817-824.
22. Fozard JR, Pfannkuche HJ, Schuurman HJ. Mast cell degranulation following adenosine A3 receptor activation in rats. *Eur J Pharmacol.* 1996;298:293-297.
23. Hannon JP, Tigani B, Williams I, Mazzoni L, Fozard JR. Mechanism of airway hyperresponsiveness to adenosine induced by allergen challenge in actively sensitized Brown Norway rats. *Br J Pharmacol.* 2001;132:1509-1523.
24. Mascali JJ, Cvietusa P, Negri J, Borish L. Anti-inflammatory effects of theophylline: modulation of cytokine production. *Ann Allergy Asthma Immunol.* 1996;77:34-38.
25. Oliver B, Tomita K, Keller A, et al. Low-dose theophylline does not exert its anti-inflammatory effects in mild asthma through upregulation of interleukin-10 in alveolar macrophages. *Allergy.* 2001;56:1087-1090.
26. Lim S, Tomita K, Caramori G, et al. Low-dose theophylline reduces eosinophilic inflammation but not exhaled nitric oxide in mild asthma. *Am J Respir Crit Care Med.* 2001;164:273-276.
27. Laube BL, Edwards AM, Dalby RN, Creticos PS, Norman PS. The efficacy of slow versus faster inhalation of cromolyn sodium in protecting against allergen challenge in patients with asthma. *J Allergy Clin Immunol.* 1998;101(4 Pt 1):475-483.
28. Morrow T. Implications of pharmacogenomics in the current and future treatment of asthma. *J Manag Care Pharm.* 2007;13:497-505.

Suggested Reading

National Asthma Education and Prevention Program. *Expert panel report 3 (EPR-3): guidelines for the diagnosis and management of asthma.* Bethesda, MD: National Heart, Lung, and Blood Institute, 2007. NIH publication no. 08-4051.

WHAT IS THE ROLE OF IMMUNOTHERAPY OR ALLERGY SHOTS IN MANAGING ASTHMA?

Lisa Forbes, MD and Jonathan M. Spergel, MD, PhD

There is a close relationship between asthma and allergy. Despite this, allergen immunotherapy has been a controversial topic in the treatment of asthma for many years, and this controversy is unlikely to be completely resolved anytime soon. Many studies have investigated the utility of allergen immunotherapy in asthma with some showing clear benefit and others showing less clear results. Immunotherapy also has a unique element of risk that needs to be considered as well. Clinicians caring for children with asthma should be aware of the pros and cons of this potential therapy because it comes up regularly as part of a comprehensive discussion of asthma management options. There also needs to be awareness of which patients may be appropriate candidates for evaluation for injection immunotherapy (Table 11-1).

It has been reported that 80% of patients with asthma have allergic rhinitis and 40% of patients with allergic rhinitis have asthma.[1] Allergen immunotherapy has been shown to ameliorate asthma symptoms and to reduce asthma medication requirements, including the need to increase medications. Patients undergoing allergen immunotherapy have been shown to be less likely to develop bronchial hyper-reactivity as well. In one study, 125 *Dermatophagoides pteronyssinus* (DPt; dust mite) allergic patients were treated with rush immunotherapy. Rush immunotherapy is a specific strategy of allergen immunotherapy that rapidly advances a patient to a maintenance level of immunotherapy. In this study, patients were evaluated for the severity of asthma by symptom-medication scores and with FEV1 measurements before and after immunotherapy. The authors observed a significant decrease in mean symptom-medication scores ($p<0.0001$) and a significant improvement of FEV1 ($p<0.0001$) compared to a control group of patients and the patients' own pre-immunotherapy evaluation. The study also found that improvement after immunotherapy is significantly related to age and severity of asthma prior to treatment. Children and patients with mild asthma demonstrated greatest improvement.[2]

Table 11-1

Patients For Whom Injection Immunotherapy for Asthma Can Be Considered

- Clear evidence of IgE-mediated asthma symptoms
- Symptoms not adequately controlled with first-line medical therapy
- Ability to adhere to the treatment regimen
- Level of medication requirement (high medication burden)
- Age of the patient
- Level of medical stability (unstable asthma is a relative contraindication)
- Reduced levels of lung function
- Clinical judgment of the provider

Table 11-2

Adverse Reactions to Injection Immunotherapy

Clinical Reactions	*Risk Factors for Severe Reactions*
• Urticaria • Rhinitis • Stridor • Wheezing • Hypotension • Anaphylaxis	• Severe asthma • Age less than 5 years

---

Data such as these sound quite promising. However, the risks of treating asthma with immunotherapy are also significant (Table 11-2). Reactions may be local or systemic and most often occur during the initial phases of treatment and almost always within 30 minutes of the injection. The risks include severe reactions to the immunotherapy, and this includes the risk of fatal anaphylaxis in one in 2 million.[3]

In a 2010 Cochrane review of studies reporting asthma symptom scores as a primary outcome, there was a significant reduction in asthma symptom scores and medication requirements. Improvements in bronchial hyper-reactivity were also noted as a rule. No consistent effect on other measures of lung function was noted across the studies in this review. While the studies varied in terms of specific antigens that were targeted and the response to immunotherapy can be dependent upon the antigen(s) being desensitized, these are fairly consistent clinical findings. In terms of side effects, this review reported that roughly one patient in 16 undergoing desensitization would develop a local adverse reaction and that one patient in nine would develop a systemic reaction of any level of severity.[4]

In most studies, a reduction in the use of asthma medications following immuno-therapy has been reported. Despite these encouraging results on clinical parameters and medication usage, the data on improvement in lung function (FEV1) do not reach statistical significance.[4] In contrast, there is a more variable effect on bronchial hyper-reactivity (BHR) that varies with the challenge agent. In general, there has been shown to be a reduction in allergen-specific bronchial hyper-responsiveness, and immunotherapy-treated patients were less likely to develop allergen-specific BHR. This is an important "proof of concept" because one would expect less reactivity to something to which a patient is being desensitized.

The Preventive Allergy Treatment (PAT) study was the first long-term prospective study to investigate whether specific immunotherapy (SIT) could prevent the development of asthma and whether the effects would persist in children with birch/grass pollen allergy as they get older. The patients in this study were treated with a 3-year course of SIT, were re-evaluated after a total of 5 years, and were followed for 10 years. A total of 147 patients were followed for 10 years (68 control subjects and 79 treatment subjects). The longitudinal statistical analysis including all subjects at 3-, 5-, and 10-year marks found that BHR in childhood increased the risk for the later development of asthma and that allergen SIT with standardized allergens can prevent the development of asthma. After 3 years of SIT with high-dose allergen-standardized allergen extracts, a 10-year follow-up analysis demonstrated a persistent long-term effect on clinical symptoms after termination of immunotherapy treatment. These investigators also showed a long-term preventative effect on the development of asthma in children with seasonal rhinoconjunctivitis.[5-7]

When patients receiving allergen-specific immunotherapy for asthma were compared to untreated controls, there was a significant reduction in symptom scores, medication usage, and BHR accompanied by an increase in lung function. One study even reported a reduction in nonspecific BHR.[2,8,9] Kohno and colleagues investigated rush immuno-therapy in eight patients with dust mite allergy-induced asthma. Both early- and late-phase bronchoconstriction after bronchial provocation with allergen were decreased (p<0.03). When compared directly with inhaled corticosteroids, symptom scores and FEV1 rose more rapidly with the inhaled corticosteroid budesonide. However, there were no standard deviations reported, and no subsequent study has been performed to validate these data.[10]

Allergen-specific immunotherapy can significantly reduce asthma symptom scores and medication requirements. Across most of the studies, medication requirements dropped. This is a clinically relevant finding. Therefore, one important goal of immuno-therapy is to reduce the medication burden that a patient is experiencing. However, there has not been a study that shows a conclusive effect on lung function. The measure of pulmonary physiology that seems to be most positively impacted is BHR. Non-specific BHR is modestly improved. The clinically important piece is the significant improvement in allergen-specific BHR. For most patients who turn to immunotherapy, specific allergen exposure can cause a rapid clinical deterioration. These results provide an encouraging option for sensitive patients with a specifically identifiable trigger.

Reduction in symptoms, medication requirements, and allergen-specific BHR present a compelling case to start immunotherapy. There are, however, well-recognized side effects of starting immunotherapy in severe asthmatics. In 3 studies, the incidence of systemic reaction was one per 1250 to one per 2206 injections. The majority of reactions were mild, and deaths due to allergen immunotherapy were extremely rare (estimates one per 1 million to one per 2 million injections).[4,11-13] Favorable outcomes of non-fatal reactions compared to fatal reactions were related to a lower severity of asthma and timely appropriate treatment of life-threatening anaphylaxis.[14]

The studies examining allergen immunotherapy are encouraging for patients with specific allergen sensitivities. However, most studies report only positive findings, and there are few studies comparing immunotherapy to conventional treatment, such as inhaled corticosteroids. In the case of treating extrinsic asthma in the presence of an unavoidable allergen, treatment with the allergen-specific extract should be used with caution. The side effects of treatment and the risks of reaction in a patient with asthma should be fully discussed with the patient. With proper monitoring postinjection and expert advice on hand, immunotherapy can be considered in patients with asthma.

Immunotherapy is used as an adjuvant to standard therapies, and this is how it is positioned in the latest asthma guidelines. Patients with asthma who are to be considered candidates for immunotherapy require appropriate evaluation, consultation, and collaboration with an allergist/immunologist for proper assessment and identification of allergic triggers. Finally, the limitations and risks of immunotherapy need to be fully discussed. Immunotherapy can reduce medication usage and symptoms, but it cannot replace inhaled corticosteroids!

References

1. Bousquet J, Khaltaev N, Cruz AA, et al. Allergic rhinitis and its impact on asthma (ARIA) 2008 update (in collaboration with the World Health Organization, GA(2)LEN and AllerGen). *Allergy*. 2008;(63 Suppl 86):8-160.
2. Bousquet J, Hejjaoui A, Clauzel AM, et al. Specific immunotherapy with a standardized *Dermatophagoides pteronyssinus* extract. II. Prediction of efficacy of immunotherapy. *J Allergy Clin Immunol*. 1988;82:971-977.
3. Abramson M, Puy R, Weiner J. Immunotherapy in asthma: an updated systematic review. *Allergy*. 1999;54:1022-1041.
4. Abramson MJ, Puy RM, Weiner JM. Allergen immunotherapy for asthma. *Cochrane Database Syst Rev*. 2010;8:CD001186.
5. Moller C, Dreborg S, Ferdousi HA, et al. Pollen immunotherapy reduces the development of asthma in children with seasonal rhinoconjunctivitis (the PAT-study). *J Allergy Clin Immunol*. 2002;109:251-256.
6. Niggemann B, Jacobsen L, Dreborg S, et al. Five-year follow-up on the PAT study: specific immunotherapy and long-term prevention of asthma in children. *Allergy*. 2006;61:855-859.
7. Jacobsen L, Niggemann B, Dreborg S, et al. Specific immunotherapy has long-term preventive effect of seasonal and perennial asthma: 10-year follow-up on the PAT study. *Allergy*. 2007;62:943-948.
8. Garcia-Ortega P, Merelo A, Marrugat J, Richart C. Decrease of skin and bronchial sensitization following short-intensive scheduled immunotherapy in mite-allergic asthma. *Chest*. 1993;103:183-187.
9. Kohno Y, Minoguchi K, Oda N, et al. Effect of rush immunotherapy on airway inflammation and airway hyperresponsiveness after bronchoprovocation with allergen in asthma. *J Allergy Clin Immunol*. 1998;102(6 Pt 1):927-934.
10. Shaikh WA. Immunotherapy vs inhaled budesonide in bronchial asthma: an open, parallel, comparative trial. *Clin Exp Allergy*. 1997;27:1279-1284.
11. Businco L, Zannino L, Cantani A, Corrias A, Fiocchi A, La Rosa M. Systemic reactions to specific immunotherapy in children with respiratory allergy: a prospective study. *Pediatr Allergy Immunol*. 1995;6:44-47.
12. Karaayvaz M, Erel F, Caliskaner Z, Ozanguc N. Systemic reactions due to allergen immunotherapy. *J Investig Allergy Clin Immunol*. 1999;9:39-44.
13. Ragusa FV, Passalacqua G, Gambardella R, et al. Nonfatal systemic reactions to subcutaneous immunotherapy: a 10-year experience. *J Investig Allergy Clin Immunol*. 1997;7:151-154.
14. Amin HS, Liss GM, Bernstein DI. Evaluation of near-fatal reactions to allergen immunotherapy injections. *J Allergy Clin Immunol*. 2006;117:169-75

WHAT OTHER MEDICATIONS MIGHT I USE TO TREAT MY PATIENTS WITH ASTHMA?

Lisa Forbes, MD and Jonathan M. Spergel, MD, PhD

Anti-inflammatory medications are the mainstay of treatment for asthma. They have been shown to increase lung function (FEV1) and decrease symptoms, exacerbation frequency, and need for rescue inhalers. There are other medications that can be used as an adjuvant to anti-inflammatory therapy.

Other Bronchodilators

The anticholinergic agent ipratropium bromide (IB; Atrovent) has an additive beneficial effect when given with beta-2 agonist bronchodilators in acute severe asthma.[1] IB has a long duration of action in the large and medium-sized airways. It competes with acetylcholine at the receptor site, attenuating the cholinergic neural signal for bronchoconstriction. By this mechanism, IB leads to a downstream relaxation of the airway smooth muscle.[2] IB has poor lipid solubility, which prevents systemic absorption and minimizes side effects. Less than 1% of the inhaled dose is absorbed systemically, and there is no evidence of patients developing drug tolerance. IB begins showing therapeutic benefits within 3 to 30 minutes of inhalational administration, and it can last up to 6 hours.[2] IB may be especially beneficial in treating viral-induced asthma, and it may be worth a clinical trial in those patients poorly responsive to beta-adrenergic bronchodilators. It has been proposed that certain viruses implicated in triggering asthma may modify the acetylcholine receptor, leading to enhanced cholinergic tone. Therefore, IB may play an important role in treating viral-induced asthma.[3] The use of IB is both safe and efficacious at high doses, and it is most efficacious in improving symptoms and preventing hospital admissions due to severe asthma exacerbations when used in the emergency room early and aggressively along with short-acting beta-2 agonist inhaled therapy.[4-7] Its use in patients admitted to the hospital and even to the intensive care unit remains less well documented, and therefore IB can often be discontinued once a patient is stabilized and admitted to the hospital for ongoing management.

Tiotropium (Spiriva) is a long-acting anticholinergic agent used as add-on therapy for adults with asthma when their disease is not well controlled on inhaled glucocorticoid therapy. In one triple-blind, placebo-controlled, 3-way cross-over design, investigators reported greater improvement in peak expiratory flow and FEV1 along with better symptom control when tiotropium was added as compared to doubling the dose of inhaled corticosteroids (ICS).[8] This agent cannot be used instead of ICS, but may be considered as an additional agent for uncontrolled asthma when patients are not controlled with ICS, leukotriene modifiers, or long-acting beta-agonists.

Mast Cell Stabilizers (The Chromones)

Mast cell stabilizers were first discovered in 1965 and developed into a treatment for allergic disease in 1975. Cromolyn sodium, an inhaled dry powder, prevents antigen-induced histamine and leukotriene release from passively sensitized lung cells by inhibiting calcium channel activation after immunoglobulin-E (IgE) cross-linking by antigen.[9-12] Cromolyn sodium reaches peak levels in 8 to 16 minutes, and the mean plasma half-life is 96 to 113 minutes. It is gone after 4 hours, and only approximately 1% is absorbed systemically.[13,14] Inhaled nedocromil has similar pharmacokinetics. Efficacy is related to delivery with either an metered-dose inhaler with a spacer or with a nebulizer, as seen with cystic fibrosis patients.[15,16] The chromones have anti-inflammatory effects in the lung and have been shown to reduce sputum and bronchial mucosal eosinophils when compared to placebo as well as salmeterol and fluticasone.[17,18] The chromones have been shown to have steroid-sparing effects without a reduction in or loss of effect, and an added benefit was demonstrated in patients inadequately controlled on inhaled steroids alone.[15,19,20] There is very little toxicity associated with use of both chromones. Hypersensitivity is very rare and usually occurs at the site of application.[21-23] Their efficacy is much lower than ICS in terms of modifying asthma symptoms or improvement of lung functions, but similar to montelukast in its efficacy.[24,25] Despite these favorable safety and efficacy data, chromones are low-potency medications, and while they remain listed as therapeutic options in the National Institutes of Health and other asthma guidelines, their use is quite limited in clinical practice.

Anti-Immunoglobulin E Therapy (Omalizumab)

Omalizumab is a humanized monoclonal antibody that binds to the fragment, crystallizable portion of the IgE molecule. Its administration results in a rapid decrease in free IgE in the serum.[26,27] There is a 99% reduction in free IgE within 2 hours of administration, and within 3 months, human basophil responsiveness was also reduced.[28] Omalizumab treatment resulted in a significant decrease in sputum tissue eosinophils in a study of 45 mild to moderate asthmatic patients.[29] However, the studies relating treatment with anti-IgE and improvement in airway hyper-responsiveness have been inconsistent. Omalizumab is indicated for patients with moderate to severe persistent allergic asthma. In phase 3 clinical trials, omalizumab reduced asthma exacerbations and had steroid-sparing effects. Most patients were able to decrease or stop the inhaled steroids. There were fewer asthma symptoms, less rescue medication usage, and improved quality of life in omalizumab-treated patients as well.[30-32] Most often, omalizumab is added to the medication regimen of poorly controlled asthma despite maximizing medical therapy. There have been reports of anaphylaxis. The frequency reported to the Food and Drug Administration was 1:1000 (0.1%). Of the 39,500 patients treated with omalizumab from June 2003 to December 2005, anaphylaxis was reported in 0.1%. Anaphylaxis can occur with any dose; therefore, patients should be monitored closely after injections and should be prescribed an epinephrine rescue device.[33] The most common side effect is a local injection site reaction. Burning, pruritis, hives, pain, redness, induration, swelling, warmth, and bruising have all been reported. Despite this, omalizumab is relatively safe and offers an alternative novel approach to treating poorly controlled individuals with allergic asthma.

Emergency Medications

In emergency situations, various medications are used in emergency departments and intensive care units, including subcutaneous epinephrine, intravenous beta-agonists (terbutaline), helium and oxygen gas mixtures (heliox), magnesium, IB, and continuously nebulized albuterol. These nonstandard rescue medications may have significant toxicity and are reserved for emergent situations and closely monitored clinical environments. A complete discussion of these agents is beyond the scope of this brief discussion.

Other Therapies Under Investigation

Research is ongoing for novel therapies in the treatment of asthma. These medications include improved corticosteroids (once a day instead of twice a day), new phosphodiesterase inhibitors with fewer side effects, or long-acting bronchodilators (once a day instead of twice a day). Other medications include biological agents active against individual molecules, including anti-IL-5, anti-TNF-alpha, anti-IL-4/13, and other anti-inflammatory molecules.

References

1. Busse WW, Lemanske RF Jr. Expert panel report 3: Moving forward to improve asthma care. *J Allergy Clin Immunol.* 2007;120:1012-1014.
2. Aaron SD. The use of ipratropium bromide for the management of acute asthma exacerbation in adults and children: a systematic review. *J Asthma.* 2001;38:521-530.
3. Corne JM, Holgate ST. Mechanisms of virus induced exacerbations of asthma. *Thorax.* 1997;52:380-389. PMCID: 1758527.
4. Schuh S, Johnson DW, Callahan S, Canny G, Levison H. Efficacy of frequent nebulized ipratropium bromide added to frequent high-dose albuterol therapy in severe childhood asthma. *J Pediatr.* 1995;126:639-645.
5. Qureshi F, Pestian J, Davis P, Zaritsky A. Effect of nebulized ipratropium on the hospitalization rates of children with asthma. *N Engl J Med.* 1998;339:1030-1035.

6. Reisman J, Galdes-Sebalt M, Kazim F, Canny G, Levison H. Frequent administration by inhalation of salbutamol and ipratropium bromide in the initial management of severe acute asthma in children. *J Allergy Clin Immunol.* 1988;81:16-20.

7. Qureshi F, Zaritsky A, Lakkis H. Efficacy of nebulized ipratropium in severely asthmatic children. *Ann Emerg Med.* 1997;29:205-211.

8. Peters SP, Kunselman SJ, Icitovic N, et al. Tiotropium bromide step-up therapy for adults with uncontrolled asthma. *N Engl J Med.* 2010;363:1715-1726.

9. Sheard P, Blair AM. Disodium cromoglycate. Activity in three in vitro models of the immediate hypersensitivity reaction in lung. *Int Arch Allergy Appl Immunol.* 1970;38:217-224.

10. Hoth M, Penner R. Depletion of intracellular calcium stores activates a calcium current in mast cells. *Nature.* 1992;355:353-356.

11. Theoharides TC, Wang L, Pang X, et al. Cloning and cellular localization of the rat mast cell 78-kDa protein phosphorylated in response to the mast cell "stabilizer" cromolyn. *J Pharmacol Exp Ther.* 2000;294:810-821.

12. Theoharides TC, Sieghart W, Greengard P, Douglas WW. Antiallergic drug cromolyn may inhibit histamine secretion by regulating phosphorylation of a mast cell protein. *Science.* 1980;207:80-82.

13. Neale MG, Brown K, Foulds RA, Lal S, Morris DA, Thomas D. The pharmacokinetics of nedocromil sodium, a new drug for the treatment of reversible obstructive airways disease, in human volunteers and patients with reversible obstructive airways disease. *Br J Clin Pharmacol.* 1987;24:493-501.

14. Neale MG, Brown K, Hodder RW, Auty RM. The pharmacokinetics of sodium cromoglycate in man after intravenous and inhalation administration. *Br J Clin Pharmacol.* 1986;22:373-382.

15. Laube BL, Edwards AM, Dalby RN, Creticos PS, Norman PS. The efficacy of slow versus faster inhalation of cromolyn sodium in protecting against allergen challenge in patients with asthma. *J Allergy Clin Immunol.* 1998;101(4 Pt 1):475-483.

16. Aswania O, Chrystyn H. Relative lung bioavailability of generic sodium cromoglycate inhalers used with and without a spacer device. *Pulm Pharmacol Ther.* 2001;14:129-133.

17. Kennedy MC. Disodium cromoglycate in the control of asthma. A double-blind trial. *Br J Dis Chest.* 1969;63:96-106.

18. Lindqvist A, Karjalainen EM, Laitinen LA, et al. Salmeterol resolves airway obstruction but does not possess anti-eosinophil efficacy in newly diagnosed asthma: a randomized, double-blind, parallel group biopsy study comparing the effects of salmeterol, fluticasone propionate, and disodium cromoglycate. *J Allergy Clin Immunol.* 2003;112:23-28.

19. Sano Y, Adachi M, Kiuchi T, Miyamoto T. Effects of nebulized sodium cromoglycate on adult patients with severe refractory asthma. *Respir Med.* 2006;100:420-433.

20. Edwards AM, Stevens MT. The clinical efficacy of inhaled nedocromil sodium (Tilade) in the treatment of asthma. *Eur Respir J.* 1993;6:35-41.

21. Cox JS, Beach JE, Blair AM, et al. Disodium cromoglycate (Intal). *Adv Drug Res.* 1970;5:115-196.

22. Clark B. General pharmacology, pharmacokinetics, and toxicology of nedocromil sodium. *J Allergy Clin Immunol.* 1993;92(1 Pt 2):200-202.

23. Foulds RA. An overview of human safety data with nedocromil sodium. *J Allergy Clin Immunol.* 1993;92(1 Pt 2):202-204.

24. Cowan DC, Hewitt RS, Cowan JO, et al. Exercise-induced wheeze: Fraction of exhaled nitric oxide-directed management. *Respirology.* 2010;15:683-690.

25. Liebke C, Sommerfeld C, Wahn U, Niggemann B. [Preventive monotherapy with montelukast versus DNCG in children with mild asthma. Results of and exploratory pilot study]. *Pneumologie.* 2001;55:231-237.

26. Brownell J, Casale TB. Anti-IgE therapy. *Immunol Allergy Clin North Am.* 2004;24:551-568, v.

27. Easthope S, Jarvis B. Omalizumab. *Drugs.* 2001;61:253-260; discussion 261.

28. MacGlashan DW Jr, Bochner BS, Adelman DC, et al. Down-regulation of Fc(epsilon)RI expression on human basophils during in vivo treatment of atopic patients with anti-IgE antibody. *J Immunol.* 1997;158:1438-1445.

29. Djukanovic R, Wilson SJ, Kraft M, et al. Effects of treatment with anti-immunoglobulin E antibody omalizumab on airway inflammation in allergic asthma. *Am J Respir Crit Care Med.* 2004;170:583-593.

30. Busse W, Corren J, Lanier BQ, et al. Omalizumab, anti-IgE recombinant humanized monoclonal antibody, for the treatment of severe allergic asthma. *J Allergy Clin Immunol.* 2001;108:184-190.

31. Milgrom H, Berger W, Nayak A, et al. Treatment of childhood asthma with anti-immunoglobulin E antibody (omalizumab). *Pediatrics.* 2001;108:E36.

32. Soler M, Matz J, Townley R, et al. The anti-IgE antibody omalizumab reduces exacerbations and steroid requirement in allergic asthmatics. *Eur Respir J.* 2001;18:254-261.

33. US Food and Drug Administration, Center for Drug Evaluation and Research. *Information for healthcare professionals: omalizumab (marketed as Xolair).* Retrieved from www.fda.gov/cder/drug/infosheets/hcp/omalizumabhcp.htm.

DO ANY ALTERNATIVE THERAPIES FOR ASTHMA HAVE PROVEN EFFICACY?

Natalie M. Hayes, DO and Aaron S. Chidekel, MD

In a word: no. Well, at least not yet.

Despite this fact, many patients and parents are curious about alternative therapies for any chronic disease, and asthma is no exception. All physicians should be aware of the reality that it is quite possible that their patients are using one or more alternative therapies. This fact needs to be explored as part of comprehensive medical management and not just comprehensive asthma management.

According to the National Center for Complementary and Alternative Medicine (NCCAM), complementary and alternative medicine (CAM) is "a group of diverse medical and health care systems, practices, and products that are generally not considered part of conventional medicine."[1] As shown in Table 13-1, different types of CAM can be subdivided into several categories: 1) natural products, such as herbal supplements; 2) mind-body medicine; and 3) manipulative and body-based practices, such as yoga, acupuncture, massage therapy, osteopathic manipulative treatment (OMT), and chiropractic manipulation.[1]

One of the challenges confronting allopathic physicians is that patients may not report their use of CAM. In addition, there are limitations to the available questionnaire studies evaluating the usage of CAM, and these data need to be evaluated with care. Similarly, there is a general lack of high-quality medical evidence about the safety and efficacy of CAM, both due to an overall lack of clinical studies and the lack of governmental regulations that require study of some nonallopathic medical treatments. There are simply very few randomized, placebo-controlled studies evaluating CAM treatments, and furthermore, some forms of CAM are by their nature very difficult to study. With these caveats in mind, some of what is known about CAM is reviewed in the following paragraphs.

A recent Cochrane review article examined manual therapy in asthma.[2] In this paper, 68 articles were evaluated through August 2004; however, only 3 randomized, controlled trials met criteria for review. Two of these studies were chiropractic, and one study looked

---

Table 13-1

Domains of Complementary and Alternative Medicine

- Mind-body interventions
  - Prayer
  - Yoga
  - Breathing exercises
- Biologically-based therapies
  - Herbs
  - Supplements
  - Other dietary products

- Energy therapies
  - Reiki
  - Magnets
- Manipulative and body-based methods
  - Chiropractic
  - Massage
  - Osteopathic manipulation
- Whole alternative medical systems
  - Acupuncture
  - Ayruveda

---

at massage therapy. One of the chiropractic studies and the massage therapy study were pediatric studies. Both chiropractic studies included a sham procedure for the control group. With the two chiropractic studies, the authors concluded there was no evidence to support the use of spinal manipulation therapy in asthma. Efficacy was unclear in the massage therapy study, and final conclusions about these therapies are not able to be drawn until there is further information according to these Cochrane reviewers.[2]

In the same Cochrane review, no studies involving OMT were included. OMT also involves physical manipulation of the patient's body in specific ways, and is designed to address somatic dysfunctions identified from an osteopathic structural examination. In August 2004, Guiney and colleagues published the results of a randomized, controlled trial involving OMT and pediatric patients.[3] Peak expiratory flow rates were the main outcome measure, and the control group received a sham OMT procedure. While this study only looked at immediate effects following OMT (n = 90) versus sham (n = 50), a significant improvement in the peak expiratory flow rates in the OMT group was seen compared to the control group. The study authors discussed that a larger trial with longer follow-up, in addition to spirometry as part of the outcome measures, was needed to further address the efficacy of OMT in pediatric asthma.

Dietary supplements, herbal medicines, vitamins, and minerals are commonly used as CAM in both adults and children. Dietary supplements are not regulated by the Food and Drug Administration (FDA) to the same standards of stability, purity, and consistency as are allopathic medications. Simply put, there are different regulations for foods and drugs, and supplements are regulated as foods. Similarly, the FDA does not evaluate health claims made by supplement manufacturers as stringently as they do for allopathic medications. Finally, there is no requirement for the manufacturers of dietary supplements to report safety concerns regarding these products. This creates an additional element of risk when these products are used. While apparently rare, contamination of dietary supplements has been reported with resultant untoward effects in both adults and children. Physicians should be aware of these differences between supplements and medications and should counsel patients, particularly parents of children, accordingly

Table 13-2

Potential Adverse Safety Factors About Supplements

1. No regulation for purity, identification, and manufacturing
2. No requirement for adverse event reporting
3. Side effects may be nonspecific
4. Perceptions of safety of a natural product
5. Physicians do not ask about CAM usage
6. Patients may be reluctant to report CAM usage

Adapted from Slifman NR, Obermeyer WR, Aloi BK, et al. Contamination of botanical dietary supplements by *Digitalis lanata*. *N Engl J Med.* 1998;379:806-811.

(Table 13-2). When buying a supplement, it is often difficult, if not impossible, to know precisely what one is buying.

As with manual therapies, studies showing efficacy of dietary supplements, herbal medicine, vitamins, and minerals are lacking. Gardiner briefly reviewed a study looking at ginkgo biloba in asthma.[4] However, this study is in Chinese, so the primary source was unable to be reviewed completely. An additional challenge to the relevance of this study is the fact that ginkgo leaf extract was used in addition to a methylprednisolone inhaler, which is not used in the United States. An additional Cochrane review analyzed fish oil in both adults and children with asthma.[5] In this review of 9 randomized, controlled trials, there was no consistent effect on five different asthma outcomes.

Survey questionnaires are frequently used to determine what patients actually do, or take, for their chronic diseases, including asthma. Slader and colleagues reviewed 17 studies that investigated the use of CAM in asthma patients.[6] In adults, acupuncture, aromatherapy, breathing techniques, herbal products, homeopathy, and yoga were most frequently used. In children, breathing techniques, diet therapy, herbal medicine, homeopathy, massage, positive therapy, physical therapy, prayer, relaxation techniques, vitamins, and minerals were used most commonly.[6] The authors concluded that 20% to 30% of adults and 50% to 60% of children with asthma had used CAM. These results are higher when compared to an initial survey Chidekel and I conducted where 79 parents of 83 children with asthma responded to a questionnaire about OMT and other CAM therapies.[7] Our results showed that only 4.8% of children had received CAM, which included Chinese herbal therapy, prayer, and yoga. However, 69.9% of the parents had received one or more types of CAM, with prayer, chiropractic, dietary supplements, and massage being the most common modalities. These differences highlight the difficulty in assessing and generalizing the results of questionnaire studies.

Clearly, it is best to ask patients directly about their interest in and usage of CAM. Frequently, parents or patients do not tell their physicians that they or their children are using CAM unless directly asked. The reasons for CAM nondisclosure are likely multifactorial, but most notably it is because the physician never asked. Other reasons for "CAM nondisclosure" have included the perception that the health care provider does not need to know and the fact that patients consider these products to be supplements and not medications per se. A final reason involves the fear of a negative or judgmental response from the physician.

A practical approach to the use of complementary and alternative medical therapies in clinical practice is to address it in a clear and non-judgmental fashion. Asking curiously whether a patient or parent has either tried CAM or if they have any questions about the potential utility of alternative therapies is often sufficient to start an open conversation. Discussing the limitations of the current research regarding CAM, the limited evidence of efficacy, and the (rare) potential for harm, particularly of drug interactions, is important. Obviously, it is critical that a patient not be taking something that is known to be harmful, shown to be contaminated due to a manufacturing problem, or, in the case of a dietary supplement, containing an ingredient to which they or their child may be allergic. It is also helpful to have the patient bring in the bottle or forward any online information about the relevant product in question. Ask for the patient or parent to be open so that they can be informed of any new information about efficacy, side effects, and interactions with prescribed allopathic medical therapies, and follow up with them at each visit. Finally, review any new safety or efficacy information about the allopathic medications that are being prescribed, and reinforce the rationale for the prescription and any plans for dosage adjustments.

While CAM therapies currently have not shown efficacy in asthma management, research is ongoing, and this could change in the near future. Research investigating manual therapies is particularly challenging, as even a sham procedure in control groups could have its own effects. However, multiple surveys document at least some level of CAM use in children with asthma. Knowing which CAM therapies, if any, your patients are using or are interested in using is pertinent information that may get missed unless patients and their families are directly asked.

References

1. National Center for Complementary and Alternative Medicine. *What is CAM?* National Center for Complementary and Alternative Medicine Web site. Retrieved from www.nccam.nih.gov. Accessed November 30, 2010.
2. Hondras MA, Linde K, Jones AP. Manual therapy for asthma. *Cochrane Database of Systematic Reviews.* 2005;2:CD001002.
3. Guiney PA, Chou R, Vianna A, Lovenheim J. Effects of osteopathic manipulative treatment on pediatric patients with asthma: a randomized controlled trial. *J Am Osteopath Assoc.* 2005;105:7-12.
4. Gardiner P, Wornham W. Recent review of complementary and alternative medicine used by adolescents. *Curr Opin Pediatr.* 2000;12:298-302.
5. Woods RK. Dietary marine fatty acids (fish oil) for asthma in adults and children. *Cochrane Database of Systematic Reviews.* 2002;3:CD001283.
6. Slader CA, Reddel HK, Jenkins CR, Armour CL, Bosnic-Anticevich SZ. Complementary and alternative medicine use in asthma: who is using what? *Respirology.* 2006;11:373-387.
7. Hayes N, Chidekel A. Comparison of knowledge and attitudes regarding osteopathic manipulative treatment and other forms of complementary and alternative medicine therapies among parents of children with cystic fibrosis and asthma. *Pediatr Pulmonol Suppl.* 2006;29:A549.

WHAT MEDICATION DELIVERY DEVICES ARE USED IN THE MEDICAL MANAGEMENT OF ASTHMA AND HOW DO THEY WORK?

David E. Geller, MD

Asthma-management guidelines stress the importance of inhaled corticosteroids and bronchodilators for controlling inflammation and symptoms. Inhaled therapy provides a high airway concentration of medication using lower doses than systemic treatment, thus maximizing the desired effects and reducing systemic effects. In the case of inhaled bronchodilators, the onset of action is far quicker than oral therapy, providing rapid relief of bronchospasm. For inhaled corticosteroids, the improved therapeutic index helps to avoid side effects of adrenal and growth suppression. However, successful aerosol delivery is much more challenging than oral or systemic drug delivery. The respiratory tract has evolved to exclude foreign materials from the lower airways. Aerosol devices and breathing techniques must be able to bypass these defenses to deposit drugs in the lungs. The proliferation of asthma drugs and devices in recent years has nurtured claims of superiority by the various manufacturers, leaving clinicians and patients confused and frustrated. Therefore, this chapter will briefly review the variables that govern aerosol deposition in the airways and the devices that deliver the drugs and will address some of the myths surrounding aerosol therapy.

Both aerosol characteristics and patient variables govern the deposition of inhaled drugs. The most important aerosol characteristic is particle size; particles less than 5 to 6 μm in size more easily navigate beyond the upper airway to reach the lungs. Velocity is the other important variable and is determined by the speed at which the particle is generated by the device and the inspiratory flow rate of the patient. Generally, smaller and slower particles have a better chance of depositing in the lower airways. Other patient variables include upper airway anatomy (which acts as a filter), disease severity (aerosols cannot penetrate beyond obstructed airways), depth of inhalation, respiratory rate, breath-holding, physical and cognitive ability to use the prescribed device, and adherence to the treatment plan.

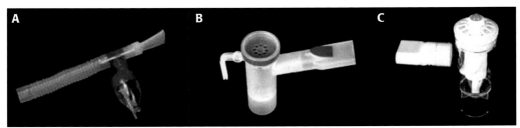

Figure 14-1. Jet nebulizer types include (A) t-piece, (B) breath-enhanced, and (C) breath-actuated (right).

Delivery devices for inhaled medications include wet nebulizers, pressurized metered-dose inhalers (pMDIs), and dry-powder inhalers (DPIs). Each of these devices has advantages and disadvantages, and because of the number of variables involved, the proportion of the nominal dose reaching the lower airways is highly variable. Fortunately, the dose-response curves for bronchodilators and inhaled corticosteroids (ICS) are steep at low doses, and because the therapeutic index is high with these drugs, the inefficiency and high variability of these delivery systems has been tolerated. More efficient systems have been developed for expensive drugs (like those used to treat cystic fibrosis), but they have not yet crossed over to the asthma realm.

Nebulizers convert a liquid solution or suspension into an aerosol. The only suspension currently available is budesonide; the available bronchodilators are in solution form. The three general types of nebulizer are the jet nebulizer, ultrasonic nebulizer, and perforated-mesh nebulizer. The jet nebulizer is the type most commonly prescribed by pediatricians, probably due to the relatively low cost and wide availability. Nebulizers are perhaps the most intuitive devices for aerosol delivery in children, as they do not require special breathing techniques (just tidal breathing) and can be used by patients of all ages. However, the delivery efficiency between nebulizer types and brands differs by several-fold and depends on design differences, airflow, and other variables. Jet nebulizers require a compressed gas source and are available in three general types: t-piece (also called "acorn" or "updraft"), breath-enhanced, and breath-actuated (Figure 14-1). The t-piece has the oldest design but is widely distributed because it is the least costly. It operates continuously, so drug is wasted during exhalation. Breath-enhanced nebulizers (eg, PARI LC or Sidestream Plus) incorporate a valve that directs inspired air through the medicine cup to capture more aerosol while inhaling and waste less while exhaling. Breath-actuated nebulizers are occasionally used in hospitals and only release aerosol during inhalation. While they are the most efficient at drug delivery, they also are more time-consuming and may result in side effects if the same nominal dose is used as with the less efficient nebulizer types.

Ultrasonic nebulizers have a piezoelectric element that transmits energy through a liquid to create an aerosol without an external gas source. They operate silently and nebulize more quickly than jet nebulizers, in general. In recent years, new models have been introduced that are smaller, more portable, and less expensive than their predecessors, and some are battery operated. However, they tend to produce a larger particle size than jet nebulizers, and they cannot effectively deliver suspension drugs (eg, budesonide). Vibrating, perforated-mesh nebulizers are the newest type and operate by oscillating a

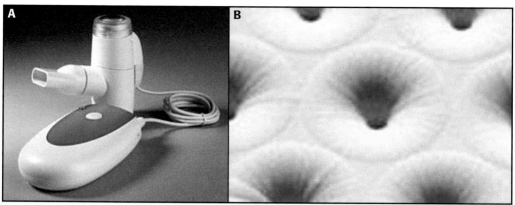

Figure 14-2. (A) A vibrating, perforated mesh nebulizer and (B) a magnified view of the mesh.

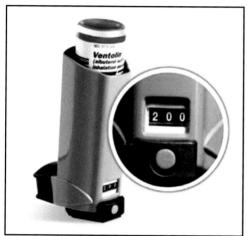

Figure 14-3. Pressurized metered-dose inhaler with dose counter.

membrane with tiny holes against a solution to "pump" the liquid through the holes, creating an aerosol (Figure 14-2). These devices are also small, silent, and fast and can be battery operated. They are still more expensive than jet nebulizers and are not recommended for suspensions because the tiny holes may get clogged with drug particles.

In general, the advantages of nebulizers include the easy technique (tidal breathing) and the ability to use them in patients of any age group and disease severity. The disadvantages include longer treatment times, requirement of a power source, and need for routine cleaning and disinfection. Nebulizers are also less portable than pMDIs and DPIs, and there are large differences in efficiency between brands. The interface between the device and child is very important as well. Until the age of 3 to 5 years, a close-fitting mask should be used. As soon as a child can use a mouthpiece, he or she should be transitioned to one to eliminate the filtering of drug that occurs with nose breathing.

Pressurized MDIs (or "puffers") are devices well suited to deliver microgram quantities of drug and are very popular because they are small, portable, and very convenient to use (Figure 14-3). A pMDI canister holds a mixture of drug (either in suspension or solution), excipients, and propellant. When the device is actuated, there is a sudden reduction of pressure in the metering chamber, causing rapid boiling of the propellant and a high-velocity release of drug over a few microseconds. In recent years, there has been a transition from chlorofluorocarbon (CFC) propellants to hydrofluoroalkanes (HFA) in order to protect the ozone layer in the atmosphere. In general, the aerosol plume from HFA pMDIs is slower and warmer than CFC predecessors, with less throat impaction and no "cold freon effect." Most of the HFA formulations produce the same particle size as the earlier CFC versions, but two of the drugs were completely reformulated as solutions instead of suspensions. As a result, both beclomethasone-HFA and ciclesonide-HFA inhalers produce a mass median particle diameter of about 1 μm. In older children and adults, this translates to about 50% of the nominal dose deposited in the lungs, far higher than other HFA or CFC inhalers. Theoretically, the smaller particles may also be an advantage in young children with smaller airways to allow deeper penetration in the lungs.

One difficulty with pMDIs is the inability to tell when the canister is empty. Many inhalers can produce a visible aerosol, even when the medication has run out. It is impossible to tell how much drug is left in the device unless one keeps track of how many doses are used. This, of course, places patients at risk for not getting any benefit from their rescue inhaler when they are symptomatic. In recent years, manufacturers have added dose counters to some of the pMDIs to address this problem, and this trend will likely continue. Also, pMDIs need to be primed when first used or when not used for a period of time (priming varies between two to four puffs after a no-use period of between 3 days to 4 weeks, depending on the drug).

Even though pMDIs have been in use for more than half a century, it is well-recognized that patients do not always use the optimal technique. Patients often make numerous errors when using pMDIs, like inhaling too rapidly or not timing the device actuation with inhalation. Many clinicians don't understand the basics of aerosol devices, so they cannot teach the technique effectively. It cannot be emphasized enough that when a pMDI is prescribed, the technique must be taught in the office by someone who is expert in the technique, and the teaching needs to be reinforced at subsequent visits. To address the issue of poor technique, numerous add-on devices (spacers and valved holding chambers [VHCs]) have been designed to allow the velocity of the plume to slow to reduce throat deposition and to improve the drug delivery to the lungs if the actuation of the device is not timed well with inspiration. VHCs with attached facemasks allow infants and toddlers to use pMDI medications, though there must be a good seal between the face and the mask in order for the medication to be delivered properly. There are many brands and types of VHCs on the market, but comparisons are difficult to do because the design features (materials, masks, valves) change frequently. Aerosol output characteristics vary greatly between devices. One of the design features that improved VHC performance significantly was the use of nonstatic plastics for the chamber, which causes less deposition inside the VHC to permit more of the drug to be delivered to the child. VHCs are recommended for use with ICS to reduce the side effects from throat deposition and for patients with poor pMDI technique. For infants and toddlers using a mask VHC, only tidal breathing is required. As comprehension improves, children can be taught the single-breath technique: 1) shake the pMDI for a few seconds, 2) exhale, 3) place the mouthpiece of the pMDI (or VHC) between the lips, 4) actuate the puffer at the beginning of a slow, deep inhalation, and 5) hold the breath for 10 seconds.

Another inhaler technology was developed that does not require the use of propellants. The Respimat Soft Mist Inhaler (Boehringer Ingelheim GmbH, Ingelheim, Germany) uses

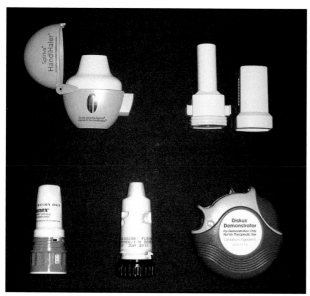

Figure 14-4. Single-dose and multi-dose dry powder inhalers.

spring-loaded mechanical energy to force the drug solution through tiny nozzles to create an aerosol that has a slower plume than the traditional pMDI. Respimat is approved in the United States for the combination of ipratropium bromide and albuterol sulfate.

DPIs use the force of the inspiratory effort to separate the powder drug into an aerosol and have the same advantages as pMDIs (ie, compact, portable, and quick to use). In addition, because they are breath-actuated, they eliminate the need for coordinating the inspiratory effort with actuation of the device. The optimal function of a DPI requires a minimum flow rate to de-agglomerate the powder and a minimum lung capacity to inhale it deeply in the lungs. Normally, children 6 years and older have the capability of using most DPIs correctly. For DPIs, the drug is milled into small, respirable particles, which tend to stick together due to strong forces of attraction. To aid separation of drug particles, often, larger (nonrespirable) particles of lactose are blended into the formulation to keep the smaller drug particles separated. Light, porous particles are being used in novel formulations to deliver large drug payloads to the lung (eg, antibiotics for CF), but asthma drugs have not yet been approved using this technology.

DPIs in general are easier to use than pMDIs, but there are many different designs (Figure 14-4), so learning how to use one type of DPI does not make it intuitive to learn a different type. Some DPIs are capsule-based, single-dose devices. A capsule containing the medication is loaded into the device chamber, where it is pierced, allowing escape of the drug as the capsule spins around during exhalation. The capsule can then be visually inspected to make sure the drug was delivered. Multi-dose DPIs either contain bulk drug in a reservoir that is metered into dosing chambers before each use or individual doses of drug that are protected by foil. Not only does the technique of loading these devices differ from one another, but they also differ in their internal resistances, making it "feel" easier or harder to inhale, depending on the device. This is not an issue for pMDIs or nebulizers. Nevertheless, many clinicians and patients prefer DPIs because of their convenience and ease of use.

There are many widely held beliefs about aerosol devices and delivery in children that deserve mention.

Myth #1: "Infants and young children are smaller, so the dose needs to be lower."
Pediatricians and family physicians treat asthma from infancy to early adulthood. Most of the aerosol variables work against infants and younger children (smaller upper and lower airway size, nasal breathing, small tidal volume, faster breathing rate), with less drug reaching the lungs. This has been shown with both nuclear scintigraphy (deposition) studies as well as pharmacokinetic studies. Yet, when the lung dose is size-corrected, deposition is similar to that of older children and adults. Unlike with oral drugs, dose-adjustment is not necessary with most inhaled therapies based on size. The overriding principle should be that the clinical response governs dose, not age or size.

Myth #2: "If a child cries during aerosol administration, he or she will get more drug in the lungs because he or she is breathing deeply."
This myth simply will not disappear! When a child cries, he or she usually inhales rapidly, then exhales (loudly) for a very long time. The rapid inhalation increases drug impaction in the throat, and more drug is wasted during a long exhalation or apneic pause. This can cause the child to reduce his or her lung dose by 75% or more. Young children should inhale medicines with relaxed, tidal breathing, using the device they tolerate the best. If they will not tolerate a mask directly on the face, our lab has shown that directing a nebulized aerosol toward the mouth and nose via corrugated tube extension works very well, but holding a mask away from the face does not work (the aerosol diffuses away from the child).

Myth #3: "I have been told that pMDIs with VHCs work much better than nebulizers (or vice versa)."
The literature is bursting with comparative studies between inhaler devices, often with conflicting results. However, comprehensive meta-analyses conclude that each of the aerosol devices works equally well in a variety of clinical settings in patients who can use the devices appropriately. That means the caregiver has the responsibility of evaluating each patient's ability to use a prescribed device and to educate him or her in the proper device techniques.

Table 14-1 shows which asthma drug formulations are available in which delivery systems in the United States. In order to help caregivers with aerosol questions, the American Association for Respiratory Care has updated a comprehensive guide on aerosol delivery, with detailed instructions for how to use, clean, and care for each device. The guide can be downloaded at www.aarc.org/education/aerosol_devices.

Choosing the "right" asthma devices for your patients is dependent on several variables. Does the device you want to use deliver the type of drug you are prescribing? Can the same device type be used for all prescribed drugs (eg, there are no rescue bronchodilators available in a DPI)? Is the device appropriate for age and capability of the child? Is it covered by third-party payers? Affordable? Convenient? Preferred and accepted by the child and the family? Having an understanding of the variables involved with aerosol therapies and devices will increase the chances for successful outcomes in asthma.

Table 14-1

Asthma Drug Formulations in the United States

	Nebulizer	pMDI	DPI (Single dose)	DPI (Multi-dose)
Short-Acting Bronchodilators				
Albuterol	✓	✓		
Lev-albuterol	✓	✓		
Pirbuterol*†		✓		
Terbutaline	✓	✓		
Ipratropium	✓	✓		
Albuterol + ipratropium†**	✓	✓		
Long-Acting Bronchodilators				
Salmeterol				✓
Formoterol	✓		✓	
Arformoterol	✓			
Tiotropium			✓	
Inhaled Corticosteroids				
Budesonide	✓			✓
Mometasone				✓
Fluticasone		✓		
Beclomethasone		✓		
Ciclesonide		✓		
Combination ICS/LABA				
Budesonide/ formoterol		✓		
Fluticasone/ salmeterol		✓		✓
Mometasone/ formoterol		✓		

*Breath-actuated pMDI; coordinates inhalation with actuation
** Approved in Respimat Soft Mist Inhaler format
†Not available as a CFC pMDI after 12/31/2013

pMDI indicates pressurized metered-dose inhalers; DPI, dry-powder inhalers; ICS, inhaled corticosteroids; LABA, long-acting beta-agonist.

Suggested Readings

Ari A, Hess D, Myers TR, Rau JL. *A guide to aerosol delivery devices for respiratory therapists.* 2nd ed. American Association for Respiratory Care, 2009. Retrieved from www.aarc.org/education/aerosol_devices.

Chua HL, Collis GG, Newbury AM, et al. The influence of age on aerosol deposition in children with cystic fibrosis. *Eur Respir J.* 1994;7:2185-2191.

Dolovich MB, Ahrens RC, Hess DR, et al. Device selection and outcomes of aerosol therapy: Evidence-based guidelines. *Chest.* 2005;127:335-371.

Geller DE. New liquid aerosol generation devices: systems that force pressurized liquids through nozzles. *Respir Care.* 2002;47:1392-1405.

Geller DE. Comparing clinical features of the nebulizer, metered-dose inhaler, and dry powder inhaler. *Respir Care.* 2005;50:1313-1322.

Hess DR. Aerosol delivery devices in the treatment of asthma. *Respir Care.* 2008;53:699-723.

Khan Y, Tang Y, Hochhaus G, et al. Lung bioavailability of hydrofluoroalkane fluticasone in young children when delivered by an antistatic chamber/mask. *J Pediatr.* 2006;149:793-797.

Labiris NR, Dolovich MB. Pulmonary drug delivery. Part I: physiologic factors affecting therapeutic effectiveness of aerosolized medications. *Br J Clin Pharmacol.* 2003;56:588-599.

Marguet C, Couderc L, Le Roux P, Jeannot E, Lefay V, Mallet E. Inhalation treatment: Errors in application and difficulties in acceptance of the devices are frequent in wheezy infants and young children. *Pediatr Allergy Immunol.* 2001;12:224-230.

National Asthma Education and Prevention Program. *Expert panel report 3 (EPR-3): guidelines for the diagnosis and management of asthma.* Bethesda, MD: National Heart, Lung, and Blood Institute, 2007. NIH publication no. 08-4051.

Self TH, Arnold LB, Czosnowski LM, Swanson JM, Swanson H. Inadequate skill of healthcare professionals in using asthma inhalation devices. *J Asthma.* 2007;44:593-598.

SECTION IV

ENVIRONMENTAL INFLUENCES

WHAT ARE THE MOST IMPORTANT ALLERGIC ASTHMA TRIGGERS?

Stephen J. McGeady, MD

The relationship between allergic disease and asthma is complicated and continues to be explored. While it is well known that asthmatic symptoms can be produced in some highly allergic subjects by allergen exposure (eg, to a dog or cat), the heterogeneous nature of asthma makes it impossible to generalize this phenomenon to all asthmatics. Despite this uncertainty, several lines of evidence point to a role for allergens in the causation of asthma, and this association seems especially strong in children. The first line of evidence is the observation that 80% of asthmatic children are skin test-positive to one or more allergens, and a similar prevalence has recently been found in adults.[1] While this association of positive skin tests and asthma is not proof of causation, it reflects a prevalence of skin test positivity that is many times that of children in general and suggests a connection. The second line of evidence derives from experimental inhalation of allergens by asthmatic subjects for research purposes. These studies have shown that inhalation of allergens to which the individual is sensitive, but not irrelevant allergens, causes the subject to experience an acute drop in forced expiratory volume in 1 second (FEV1), referred to as an early asthmatic response (EAR). This early response may be followed in several hours by a late asthmatic response (LAR) consisting of a similar drop in FEV1.[2] The allergen challenge is usually followed by a period of bronchial hyper-reactivity (BHR) to inhaled histamine or methacholine that may last several weeks[3] and is similar to BHR seen in poorly controlled asthma. The final piece of evidence is the finding of increased numbers of eosinophils and basophils in broncho-alveolar lavage fluid or in sputum following allergen inhalation challenge of asthmatic patients. Because airway eosinophilia is often found in asthmatic subjects, allergen provocation is able to reproduce this marker as well,[4] giving evidence of comparable immunopathology. In summary, inhalation of allergens in allergic subjects with asthma reproduces the bronchospasm, BHR, and airway hypereosinophilia that are the hallmarks of bronchial asthma. Together with the skin test observations, this evidence strongly supports a role for allergens in at least those asthmatics who are allergic. The importance of exposure to inhaled allergens has been considered for both indoor allergens, most likely to be encountered in the home, and outdoor allergens. The indoor allergens have been found to be the most important in allergic asthma. The reasons for the greater importance of indoor allergens are the large amount of time spent indoors, especially in the home, and the confined indoor environment, which permits buildup of greater concentrations of the relevant allergens.[5] In contrast, less time is spent outdoors, and the allergens encountered tend to be seasonal ones, such as pollens and molds, which are present only at certain times of year and are more likely to produce upper respiratory symptoms than asthma.

Indoor allergens are also referred to as perennial allergens because they are present regardless of season. Those most often implicated in asthma include allergens generated from animals intentionally kept as pets, arthropods such as house dust mites (HDM) and cockroaches, mice and rats, which infest some homes, and molds, which may proliferate in the home if there is excessive moisture. There is considerable evidence that these allergens play an important role both as causes of asthma and in triggering asthma exacerbations in sensitized individuals.[6-8] HDM are thought to be the most important indoor allergen causing asthma in temperate climates and have been the focus of many studies on the role of allergens in asthma. In one report, the authors looked prospectively at a cohort of 67 children at risk for developing asthma based on their family history. Of the 16 children who had developed active asthma at age 11 years, all but one had positive skin tests to HDM, and all those afflicted had been exposed to a high level of HDM allergen in their homes, as shown by house dust samples that were collected from the homes when the children were 1 year of age. This finding led the authors to conclude that development of asthma, while influenced by genetic factors, is contributed to by exposure to high levels of HDM allergen.[9] Other studies have noted that there are geographic and socioeconomic differences in the frequency of sensitization to HDM. It has been found that in locations where the climate is arid, such as at high altitudes, or in cold regions where artificial heating of the home is prolonged for much of the year, the prevalence of asthma remains as elsewhere, but HDM cannot survive and, consequently, HDM sensitization is diminished among asthmatics. Other allergens, such as animal emanations, are more prevalent sensitizers.[10] It has also been found among asthmatic children living in the inner cities in impoverished conditions that the prevalence of sensitivity to cockroaches and molds exceeds that to HDM, although all are prevalent.[11] Domestic animals are often sources of allergen as well, and because the particles that contain the animals' allergenic material are very small and light, they may remain airborne for long periods of time. This characteristic of animal allergens is quite different from the allergenic particles of HDM and cockroach, which are larger and heavier and tend to settle quickly rather than remaining airborne. Molds are most likely to be present in large amounts in water-damaged buildings. The spores of molds are highly airborne and may be allergenic. Recent research has suggested that molds may act as triggers of allergic or asthmatic events and incite new cases of asthma[12]; however, because they require moisture to survive, their relevance is limited to water-damaged or water-containing buildings. A recent survey of 830 housing units located in 75 different locations throughout the United States assayed levels of HDM, dog, cat, cockroach, mouse, and mold allergens. The survey found that 46% of homes had elevated levels of at least three allergens, suggesting that multiple indoor allergen exposure is commonplace and might contribute to asthma more than single allergens.[13]

Outdoor or seasonal allergens, as noted above, have not been implicated in causing or inciting asthma to the same degree as the indoor allergens. Some asthmatics describe a seasonal pattern to their symptoms or have asthma exacerbations that coincide with the appearance of seasonal allergens, such as grass or ragweed pollens, but attempts to implicate the seasonal allergens as direct causes of asthmatic symptoms have been difficult, and the association is less certain. An example of this difficulty is a study of adult asthmatics who were treated with allergen immunotherapy to ragweed extract because of a history consistent with seasonal asthma. The study could identify only minimal improvement in the ragweed-treated subjects compared with placebo-treated control subjects.[14] An editorial discussing this study noted that the investigators needed to screen 1000 subjects to identify 77 who had symptoms that clearly coincided with ragweed pollen exposure.[15] A possible association of *Alternaria* mold spores with respiratory arrest in asthmatics has been reported, with these events taking place in the summer and early fall when *Alternaria* spore counts are high. The study was retrospective and did not show actual spore counts, however.[16]

Summary

It is indoor exposure to allergens that are perennially present that seems most correlated with asthma. The most important of these are allergens associated with HDM, cat, dog, cockroach, mold, and rodents.

References

1. Craig TJ, King TS, Lemanske RF Jr, et al. Aeroallergen sensitization correlates with PC(20) and exhaled nitric oxide in subjects with mild-to-moderate asthma; National Heart, Lung, and Blood Institute's Asthma Clinical Research Network. *J Allergy Clin Immunol*. 2008;121:671-677.
2. De Monchy JG, Kauffman HF, Venge P, et al. Bronchoalveolar eosinophilia during allergen-induced late asthmatic reactions. *Am Rev Respir Dis*. 1985;131:373-376.
3. O'Byrne PM, Dolovich J, Hargreave FE. Late asthmatic responses. *Am Rev Respir Dis*. 1987;136:740-751.
4. Wardlaw AJ, Brightling CE, Green R, Woltmann G, Bradding P, Pavord ID. New insights into the relationship between airway inflammation and asthma. *Clin Sci (Lond)*. 2002;103:201-211.
5. Leech JA, Nelson WC, Burnett RT, Aaron S, Raizenne ME. It's about time: a comparison of Canadian and American time-activity patterns. *J Expo Anal Environ Epidemiol*. 2002;12:427-432.
6. Committee on the Assessment of Asthma and Indoor Air, Division of Health Promotion and Disease Prevention, Institute of Medicine. *Clearing the Air: Asthma and Indoor Exposures*. Washington, DC: National Academy Press; 2000.
7. Platts-Mills TA, Vervloet D, Thomas WR, Aalberse RC, Chapman MD. Indoor allergens and asthma: report of the Third International Workshop. *J Allergy Clin Immunol*. 1997;100(6 Pt 1):S2-S24.
8. Langley SJ, Goldthorpe S, Craven M, Morris J, Woodcock A, Custovic A. Exposure and sensitization to indoor allergens: association with lung function, bronchial reactivity, and exhaled nitric oxide measures in asthma. *J Allergy Clin Immunol*. 2003;112:362-368.
9. Sporik R, Holgate ST, Platts-Mills TA, Cogswell JJ. Exposure to house-dust mite allergen (Der p I) and the development of asthma in childhood. A prospective study. *N Engl J Med*. 1990;323:502-507.
10. Ploschke P, Janson C, Norman E, et al. Association between atopic sensitization and asthma and bronchial hyperresponsiveness in Swedish adults: Pets not mites are the most important allergens. *J Allergy Clin Immunol*. 1999;103:58-65.
11. Eggleston PA. The environment and asthma in US inner cities. *Chest*. 2007(5 Suppl);132:782S-785S.
12. Jaakkola J, Hwang BF, Jaakkola N. Home dampness and molds, parental atopy and asthma in childhood: a six-year population-based cohort study. *Environ Health Perspect*. 2005;113:357-361.

13. Salo PM, Arbes SJ Jr, Crockett PW, Thorne PS, Cohn RD, Zeldin DC. Exposure to multiple indoor allergens in US homes and its relationship to asthma. *J Allergy Clin Immunol.* 2008;121:678-684, e2.
14. Creticos PS, Reed CE, Norman PS, et al. Ragweed immunotherapy in adult asthma. *N Engl J Med.* 1996;334:501-506.
15. Barnes PJ. Is immunotherapy for asthma worthwhile? *N Engl J Med.* 1996;334:531-532.
16. O'Hollaren MT, Yunginger JW, Offord KP, et al. Exposure to an aeroallergen as a precipitating factor in respiratory arrest in young patients with asthma. *N Engl J Med.* 1991;324:359-363.

Is Environmental Tobacco Smoke Really That Bad for My Patients With Asthma?

Aaron S. Chidekel, MD and Sheela Raikar, MD

The short answer is yes. Smoking and environmental tobacco or secondhand smoke exposure is bad for everyone, but, among people with asthma, the combination is particularly toxic.

Asthma is the most common chronic disease among children in the United States, and tobacco smoking is still very common in western countries. Asthma continues to be a leading cause of missed school days, emergency department visits, and hospitalizations among children, and smoking remains a leading cause of death and disease. Uncontrolled asthma, in general, leads to difficulty with exercise, sleep, and participating in normal activities of childhood, and secondhand smoke exposure is an important contributor to uncontrolled asthma. Asthma is a chronic lung disease that is characterized by inflammation of the airway, airway hyper-responsiveness to various stimuli such as viruses, allergens, and tobacco smoke, and lower airway obstruction that is reversible, and smoking is an obvious cause of lung disease. Elimination of an important trigger or causative agent of asthma, such as tobacco smoke, represents a crucial target for intervention, just as elimination of tobacco as a threat to human health has been an important public health goal for decades. Indeed, preventing toxic tobacco smoke exposure can lead to a significant decrease in the morbidity and mortality associated with asthma and can serve to generally decrease the burden of asthma to our patients and to society. The same would be true to society at large if our country could ever truly eliminate the same problems associated with primary smoking.

Environmental tobacco smoke (ETS) is an incredibly complex substance. It is composed of side-stream smoke that is released from a lit cigarette and mainstream smoke that is exhaled by an active smoker. Because side-stream smoke burns at a lower temperature and has not been "prefiltered" by the smoker, it tends to be more toxic and irritating. Tobacco smoke has been described as a veritable "toxic brew" that contains more than

4000 chemical compounds, of which at least 43 are known carcinogens. It is classified by the EPA, along with radon and asbestos, as a Class A toxin, or a substance known to cause human disease. Condensates of tobacco smoke when applied to the skin of mice cause carcinomas and papillomas at the site of application, and components of tobacco smoke cause breaks in human DNA. One of the most notorious carcinogens in tobacco smoke is Benzo (A) Pyrene, which has been shown in the laboratory to induce gene mutations in airway epithelial cells that mimic those found in human lung carcinomas.

Data regarding smoking rates and tobacco smoke exposure are tracked closely by the governments of most westernized countries. While the numbers are fluid, smoking rates and the rates of ETS exposure among children and pregnant women remain stubbornly high. According to recent statistics, approximately 25% of the population in the United States smokes cigarettes. Tobacco use among adolescents, including those with asthma, is at best stable in the United States at around 20%. Extrapolated to the population at large, these data suggest that approximately 6 million teenagers smoke habitually, including 100,000 children under the age of 13. Further extrapolation of these data leads to the even more disturbing fact that 3000 teenagers begin to smoke each day.

Smoking rates are also heavily dependent upon sociodemographic factors. In general, smoking rates are highest among people with the least amount of education and among individuals with lower income levels. This fact has led to the promotion of increased tobacco sales taxes as an effective means of decreasing smoking initiation among cost-sensitive teens. Smoking rates also vary among different ethnic groups, indicating that physicians should be aware of those groups in their practices that are particularly at risk.

As smoking has become more socially acceptable among women, it is not surprising that tobacco smoke exposure among children is common. For example, approximately a quarter of fetuses are exposed to tobacco smoke due to maternal smoking, and because women are more likely than men to be the primary caregivers of children, maternal smoking is of particular concern when considering the exposure of children. Because children living in temperate climates spend more than half of their time indoors, the contribution of ETS to indoor air pollution is enormous.

Demonstrating the health effects of primary smoking was complicated and contentious, and what now seems obvious was often the subject of previous debate. It took a long time for the undeniable health effects of primary smoking to become accepted. It is not surprising, therefore, that the evolution of the knowledge about the adverse effects of ETS exposure has been similarly lengthy and at times controversial. Cause and effect remains very difficult to prove, even in large epidemiological studies, but the strong statistical association between adverse health effects and ETS exposure remains incredibly consistent. This is true across the life of a child beginning in utero. In general, prenatal exposure has been linked most strongly to the risk of developing asthma, whereas postnatal smoke exposure is most strongly linked with frequency and severity of respiratory symptoms and infections. ETS exposure is also a strong risk factor for sudden infant death syndrome (SIDS). Importantly, in many studies, a dose-effect has been demonstrated as well, whereby increased smoking rates as measured by the number of cigarettes smoked per day have been associated with worse health outcomes.

It has been demonstrated in many studies that ETS exposure during fetal life has multi-system effects that contribute to decreased health postnatally. Maternal smoking during pregnancy causes decreased infant pulmonary function, most likely due to effects on lung growth and development. Studies have shown effects on fetal immunity as indicated by increased levels of cord blood immunoglobulin-E (IgE) and immunoglobulin-D (IgD). There is also an increased risk of developing atopy in the first 2 years of life due to maternal smoking during pregnancy. Significantly, it is infants without a family history of atopy who had the highest risk of developing allergic symptoms in these studies. Data such as these have major implications for the development of asthma due to the important link between asthma and atopy.

In addition to these effects in fetal life, ETS exposure postnatally has a major impact on the respiratory health of infants and children as well. The risk of developing asthma is significantly increased in children exposed to tobacco smoke. One study of more than 4000 children found that children whose mothers smoked more than 10 cigarettes per day had increased odds ratios for developing asthma, for the need for asthma medications, and for the development of asthma in the first year of life. ETS exposure is believed to cause up to 26,000 cases of asthma each year, resulting in up to 1.8 million physician visits and 14 deaths annually. When compared to children who are not exposed to ETS, children exposed to tobacco smoke have increased hospitalization rates for asthma, have decreased levels of measured lung function, and have increased levels of bronchial hyperresponsiveness at all ages, including infancy. Children with asthma who are exposed to ETS have increased need for asthma medication and higher levels of health utilization. Obviously, ETS exposure causes other problems as well. The most common respiratory symptoms that are attributed to ETS exposure include wheezing and cough, and ETS exposure is linked to increased rates of respiratory tract infections, such as otitis media and bronchitis.

Recent studies have begun to evaluate the danger of third-hand smoke. This is the residue of smoking that is found on the clothing or hair and skin of a smoker and on the furniture or in the car where people have been using tobacco products. This is another important form of toxic smoking by-products from which patients with asthma (and all children) should be protected. If parents must smoke, in addition to smoking outdoors, it is recommended that they wear a smoking jacket that can be removed and wash their hands and face to minimize exposure to harmful smoking residues on their clothing and skin.

So, now that we have established that ETS is bad for patients with asthma, what can we, as pediatricians, do about it? See Table 16-1 for some office-based strategies. Clinical practice guidelines exist to assist in assessing and counseling parents and patients about the dangers of smoking and to assist with effective and efficient interventions as well. The first step is to screen all patients with a diagnosis of asthma for exposure to ETS at every visit. The simple act of asking this question at repeated visits makes it an important issue pertaining to the patient's health. This may lead parents or other caregivers to contemplate smoking cessation. Providing education about the harmful effects of ETS is important as is advising parents who are not willing or ready to quit to only smoke outside and never in the car with or without the child present. Basically, all adults should provide clean, smoke-free air for their children to breathe and should view this as a basic necessity like food or water. Sometimes, smoking outdoors can be an important first step for parents to cut down on their own tobacco use or even a means of quitting. Breastfeeding can also be an important motivator for a new mother to quit smoking. All pediatric health care providers must discuss the dangers of smoking with their patients beginning at a young

---

Table 16-1

Office-Based Strategies for Tobacco Control

- Non (anti)-smoking clinical environment
- Involve all members of the office team in efforts
- Office tobacco coordinator
- Chart prompts for recurrent, frequent intervention
- Systematic, age-appropriate anticipatory guidance
- Chart flags of smoking patients or families
- Provide educational and quitting resources

Adapted from Feinson J, Chidekel A. Strengthening tobacco-related messages relayed in pediatric offices in Delaware: results of a pilot intervention. *Clin Ped.* 2006;45:79-82.

Table 16-2

Immediate Benefits of Stopping Smoking (Or Not Starting to Smoke)

- Improved asthma control
- Improved sense of taste and smell
- More money to spend on other things
- Better smelling breath, clothes, and hair
- Improved athletic performance
- Improved sense of well-being
- Reduced risk of skin wrinkling

---

age, realizing that the peak age of smoking experimentation and initiation is between 11 and 13 years of age. Adolescents, and particularly those with asthma, should be counseled particularly strongly about the immediate dangers of smoking to their own health (Table 16-2).

The "five-A method" should be used to assist the smoker in quitting: ask, advise, assess, assist, and arrange (Table 16-3). Ask about tobacco use in a standardized method at all visits. Be careful to be nonjudgmental, but consistent and firm. Advise all smokers to quit in a clear and strong manner. Then, assess their willingness to make an attempt at quitting. If they are truly ready, then assist them by formulating a quit plan. The quit plan may include setting a quit date, informing family members of the decision, and removing all tobacco products from the household. Provide the smoker with counseling, resources such as the national stop smoking quitline, and other local resources for support. You may also recommend the use of medications to assist in smoking cessation. And, last but not least, arrange for follow-up. As a pediatrician or family practitioner, you may refer

---

Table 16-3
The Five-As of Tobacco Counseling

1. **Ask:** Identify all tobacco users or tobacco-exposed children at every visit.
   - Employ a universal identification system, such as
     - Expanded vital signs
     - Chart flagging
     - Apply to every patient at every visit
2. **Advise:** Strongly urge all tobacco users to quit or to provide a smoke-free zone for their children.
   - Counsel in a clear, strong, and personalized manner.
   - State that quitting is important and relevant to their own or their child's health.
3. **Assess:** Determine willingness to make a quit attempt.
   - Ask if the smoker is willing to make a quit attempt now or in the near future.
   - If unwilling, consider providing additional education or intervention.
4. **Assist:** Assist the patient in quitting in one of several ways.
   - Help the patient with a quit plan.
   - Refer to a quitline.
   - Provide additional support and information as able.
5. **Arrange:** Schedule follow-up contact.
   - In pediatrics, this can be individualized to the circumstance:
     - Follow-up phone call
     - Ask at next visit about the quit attempt

Adapted from Fiore M, Bailey W, Cohen S. *Treating Tobacco Use and Dependence. Clinical Practice Guideline.* Rockville, MD: US Department of Health and Human Services. Public Health Service; 2000.

---

the smoker to his or her primary-care provider for additional support and pharmacologic assistance. One simple and effective intervention involves simply asking a parent who smokes about quitting and referring him or her to a quitline. This simple, 2-step process greatly increases the likelihood of a smoker to call a quitline as the first step in the quitting process.

Summary

Smoking remains a major public health problem, and it is a particular threat to vulnerable patients with asthma. It is clear that ETS exposure is harmful to all children across their lifespan and is a modifiable environmental factor that can have a major positive impact on the health of a child when eliminated from the asthma equation. All health care providers should be familiar with counseling and advising parents and children about the dangers of smoking. This is a topic that can be addressed efficiently and effectively with resources that are readily available and by employing best-practice techniques that are evidence based. All children should live in smoke-free zones, and the messages sent by health care providers should be clear and consistent: Smoking and smoke exposure is bad for everyone, and it is even worse for those with asthma or other respiratory conditions.

Suggested Readings

DiFranza JR, Aligne CA, Weitzman M. Prenatal and postnatal environmental tobacco smoke exposure and children's health. *Pediatrics*. 2004;113:1007-1015.

DiFranza JR, Lew RA. Morbidity and mortality in children associated with the use of tobacco products by other people. *Pediatrics*. 1996;97:560-568.

Feinson J, Chidekel A. Adult smoking and environmental tobacco smoke: a persistent health threat to children. A CME-approved article for physicians. *Delaware Medical Journal*. 2006;78:213-218.

Fiore M, Bailey W, Cohen S. *Treating Tobacco Use and Dependence. Clinical Practice Guideline*. Rockville, MD: US Department of Health and Human Services. Public Health Service; 2000.

WHAT IS THE ROLE OF VIRAL INFECTIONS IN PEDIATRIC ASTHMA?

Joel D. Klein, MD, FAAP and Jennifer LeComte, DO

Asthma is a multifactorial disease that results from a combination of genetic, immunologic, and environmental factors that influence the expression and progression of the condition. Viral infections have been a large component of the environmental factors. Many studies have attempted to define and identify the role of viruses in the inception of asthma, as well as their contribution to the frequency and severity of asthma exacerbations once the diagnosis has been established. Advances in more sensitive molecular techniques have improved the rates of viral detection in acute wheezing episodes. Prospective studies have shown that up to 90% of asthma exacerbations are caused by viral infections. More specifically, respiratory syncytial virus (RSV) and human rhinovirus (HRV) are the most commonly identified viruses associated with wheezing episodes in children and are often cited as the trigger for many asthma exacerbations (Table 17-1).

About 30% of infants will have one episode of wheezing within their first year of life. Lower respiratory tract infection associated with wheezing early in life is a risk factor for recurrent wheezing later in childhood and thus increases the risk for the subsequent development of asthma. Bronchiolitis is the most common wheezing illness that presents in infancy. RSV has been identified as the causative virus in about 70% of episodes of bronchiolitis. Children hospitalized for RSV-bronchiolitis are particularly at increased risk of recurrent respiratory problems, including asthma. Current theories postulate that RSV promotes a cell-mediated defense that stimulates an acute inflammatory process by infecting respiratory epithelial cells. Some studies have suggested that, for those who go on to have persistent asthma, RSV prevents the initiation of an effective antiviral immune response including inhibiting cytokine production. RSV also has a direct effect on the airway epithelium, resulting in airway edema, epithelial shedding, and increased mucous production, ultimately causing airway obstruction. While studies have shown that RSV infections have had a substantial impact on the risk of recurrent wheezing, the episodes

---

Table 17-1

Viral Infections Shown to Be Important Contributors to Pediatric Asthma Exacerbations

- Respiratory syncytial virus
- Human rhinovirus
- Coronavirus
- Polyomavirus
- Bocavirus
- Para-influenza
- Influenza
- Human metapneumovirus

---

of wheezing appear to decrease with age. Other factors may play a greater role in the development of persistent asthma.

HRV infections were assumed to be limited to the upper airways. However, recent data have demonstrated associations between lower respiratory infections from HRV and the development of asthma. Several studies have found that HRV was the most common virus identified in association with childhood asthma exacerbations. There are many theories about the mechanism, which includes impairment of viral clearance and, therefore, increased replication of the virus in the bronchial cells. More specifically, studies have found that HRV suppresses the interferon (IFN) response in atopic patients. The IFN response has an important role in innate antiviral immunity, and deficiency of this response results in impaired viral clearance. HRV-associated wheezing illnesses during the first 3 years of life were associated with an almost 10-fold increase in asthma risk by age 6 years in one cohort study. In that study, it was also noted that HRV-associated wheezing illness was a better indicator of asthma risk than RSV-associated wheezing.

Viral infections, however, are not the sole contributor to wheezing and exacerbations of asthma. Viral infections and history of allergies synergistically enhance the risk of wheezing. Several studies have addressed the potential consequences of the interactions between viral infections and allergic inflammation. Atopic patients with asthma have been shown to be more susceptible to respiratory infections and may develop more severe manifestations of viral respiratory infections. Several mechanisms have been proposed, including virus-induced damage to the barrier function of the airway epithelium that causes increased exposure and enhanced absorption of aero-allergens. The increased permeability of the mucosa facilitates allergen contact with the immune system. There are also studies that have shown an amplification of the inflammatory response with viral and allergen interactions.

There is a controversial theory called the "Hygiene Hypothesis" that suggests that some viral or bacterial infections might protect against the subsequent development of allergies and asthma. Support for this theory has been demonstrated in some investigations where repeated exposure to infectious diseases, such as those occurring in day-care settings, may reduce the risk of allergen sensitization. However, more evidence is needed to validate this theory.

As a direct result of more sensitive methods of viral testing, many other viruses have been implicated in wheezing illnesses. Coronavirus, adenovirus, polyomavirus, and bocavirus have been identified in wheezing illnesses, but their roles in the development of asthma are still being defined, and further studies are needed. Para-influenza, influenza, and metapneumoviruses have also been identified, but are less likely to cause wheezing in infants.

Seasonal variations of viral illnesses also play a role in pediatric asthma. RSV, metapneumoviruses, and influenza illnesses are usually limited to the winter and early spring. HRV infections occur in the spring and fall, but can occur throughout the year. Seasonal epidemiologic analyses have shown that infantile wheezing illnesses during HRV season or peak RSV seasons are important predictors of the development of persistent wheezing and asthma.

There are still questions that remain as to whether early-life viral respiratory infections cause childhood asthma by a direct result of the viral infection itself or whether the virus triggers changes in an already susceptible host. Understanding the role of viruses and how they interplay with the genetic, immunologic, and environmental factors of the patient who wheezes will allow for the development of more effective approaches to the prevention and treatment of virus-induced wheezing illnesses and ultimately strategies for the primary prevention of asthma.

Suggested Readings

Gern JE. Viral respiratory infection and the link to asthma. *Ped Infect Dis J*. 2004;23:S78-S86.

Gern JE, Lemanske RF. Infectious triggers of pediatric asthma. *Ped Clin North Am*. 2003;50:555-575.

Jackson DJ, Gangnon RE, Evans MD, et al. Wheezing rhinovirus illnesses in early life predict asthma development in high-risk children. *Am J Respir Crit Care Med*. 2008;178:667-672.

Kloepfer KM, Gern JE. Virus/allergen interactions and exacerbations of asthma. *Immunol Allergy Clin N Am*. 2010;30:553-563.

ARE THERE OTHER INFECTIONS THAT ARE IMPORTANT?

Joel D. Klein, MD, FAAP and Jennifer LeComte, DO

Any infection that can cause a respiratory illness may play a role in pediatric asthma. Viral illnesses have been most commonly identified in the inception and exacerbation of asthma in pediatrics and were addressed in Question 17. Recent studies in both children and adults suggest that infections with the atypical bacteria, in addition to viral infections, may contribute to asthma exacerbation rates and disease chronicity and severity (Table 18-1). *Chlamydia pneumoniae* and *Mycoplasma pneumoniae* are most commonly implicated. *Chlamydia* is an intracellular pathogen contrasted with *Mycoplasma*, which is an extracellular pathogen. Both attack airway epithelial cells and cause cellular damage that can result in ciliary dysfunction. Atypical bacterial infections may have similar mechanisms related to airway inflammation as viral infections. Chronic infections with *Chlamydia* or *Mycoplasma* likely promote ongoing airway inflammation that increases susceptibility to other exacerbating stimuli, such as viruses, allergens, or both. Studies have supported the potential interaction between infection and allergen sensitization by showing that tissue biopsies in patients with asthma and polymerase chain reaction (PCR)-positive evidence of *C pneumoniae* or *M pneumoniae* had greater mast cell infiltrations than those with negative PCR results.

Hahn and colleagues were the first to speculate that repeat or chronic infection with *Chlamydia* may cause asthma.[1] The study showed that there was a statistically significant association of *Chlamydia* exposure and the diagnosis of asthmatic bronchitis in the 6-month period after the onset of an acute lower respiratory tract illness. Other studies have found higher levels of *C pneumoniae*-specific antibodies in patients with asthma compared with healthy control subjects. Persistence of the *C pneumoniae* organism was more common in children with a greater frequency of exacerbations. Lieberman and colleagues studied adult patients who were hospitalized for an acute asthma exacerbation. *M pneumoniae* was isolated in 18% of patients with asthma compared to only 3% of the

Table 18-1

Causes of Atypical Pneumonia in Childhood

Infectious:	Noninfectious:
• *Mycoplasma pneumoniae* • *Chlamydia pneumoniae* • *Bordetella pertussis* • *Chlamydia psittaci* • *Mycobacterium tuberculosis* • *Histoplasma* species • *Coccidiodes* species	• Hypersensitivity pneumonitis • Inflammatory lung disease • Toxic pneumonitis

control group.[2] Data from a study from Biscardi and colleagues demonstrated about 50% of children with their first asthma attack were seropositive for *M pneumoniae*.[3] Martin and colleagues also found atypical bacteria in 50% of chronic, stable asthmatics who had no exacerbation within 3 months after bronchoscopy.[4] In this small study, 23 patients with asthma were found to be PCR-positive for *M pneumoniae* compared to one positive in the control group. Seven asthmatic patients were positive for *C pneumoniae* compared to zero in the control group. In the study, 50% were seropositive for *Chlamydia* (similar to the general population) though no *C pneumoniae* was detected in the airways of the controls. *Mycoplasma* serology was negative for all patients, despite the detection of *M pneumoniae* in the airways of 23 asthmatic patents.

Defining and clarifying the role of *Chlamydia* and *Mycoplasma* in the onset of asthma has been difficult for many reasons. While *Mycoplasma* and *Chlamydia* are less common in young children, infection with these organisms dramatically rises in school-aged children, and more than 50% of patients worldwide are seropositive for *C pneumoniae* antibodies by adulthood. Studies to confirm and expand upon the hypotheses have been impeded due to the lack of definitive serologic markers to document current or past infection, as well as the inherent difficulties in obtaining biologic specimens from the lower airway to confirm the presence of these infectious agents. Standard seromarkers are not always present in those who have a positive culture. Pathogens are rarely isolated from sputum samples and often require invasive procedures to obtain appropriate samples.

Given the association between atypical bacterial infections and asthma, one has to look at the role of antibiotics in preventing asthma or at least decreasing exacerbations. While treatment with antibiotics has shown some improvement with respect to lung function, persistence of the atypical organisms has been documented after clinical cure. Some have speculated that the antibiotics, more specifically some macrolides, have immuno-modulatory properties, including anti-inflammatory effects that contribute to the clinical improvement. Others suggest that a decrease in organism load may result in decreased cytokine production and, therefore, decreased inflammation. It has not been clear in studies that eradication of the organism is the reason for the improvement. A Cochrane review of macrolide usage in chronic asthma was limited due to very few patients, but did lean toward improvement in symptoms and eosinophilic markers of inflammation.[5]

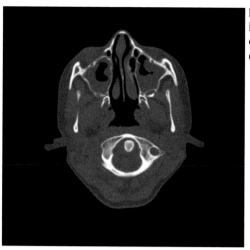

Figure 18-1. Typical computed tomography (CT) image demonstrating extensive mucosal thickening of the maxillary sinuses in a patient with difficult-to-control asthma.

Further studies are necessary to determine which patients may benefit from therapy, the timing and duration of therapy, and the optimum antibiotic. While macrolide antibiotics are occasionally used to treat refractory asthma, it is important not to over-treat asthmatic patients with antibiotics either, and there is evidence that this is sometimes the case. Appropriate use of antibiotics is a fine balance in patients with rhinitis and rhinosinusitis, but the same rules apply to asthmatic and nonasthmatic patients in terms of judicious use of antimicrobials.

Pertussis, caused by *Bordetella pertussis*, is an acute respiratory infection that is primarily a toxin-mediated disease. The bacteria attach to the cilia of the respiratory epithelial cells, produce toxins that paralyze the cilia, and cause inflammation of the respiratory tract, which interferes with the clearing of pulmonary secretions. Pertussis antigens appear to allow the organism to evade host defenses. While infants younger than 12 months with pertussis are more likely than older age groups to have complications or be hospitalized during their illness, the recent rise in pertussis in the adolescent age group may result in an exacerbation of asthma symptoms. Given the increasing incidence of pertussis, the combination of tetanus, diphtheria, and pertussis vaccine (Tdap), a vaccine with a pertussis booster, has been recommended for the adolescent age group. Tdap and other vaccines (discussed in Question 44) may minimize the effect of certain infections on asthma.

There have been some studies evaluating the association between sinusitis and asthma in children. Pathogens such as *Moraxella catarrhalis* have been identified in the sinus cultures of children both with and without asthma. Chronic pulmonary aspiration of the contents of inflamed sinuses may contribute to the cascade of airway hyper-responsiveness and ultimately lead to asthma. Treatment with antibiotics and nasal lavage appears to improve respiratory symptoms and may improve asthma control, and sinusitis is generally accepted to be an important asthma co-morbidity (Figure 18-1).

Molds including *Aspergillus* and *Mucor* have also been implicated in asthma exacerbations. Many are implicated in the host's response to allergens. Although there are many types of molds, only a few dozen cause allergic reactions. More studies are needed to identify the specific role of molds in asthma.

While it is clear that respiratory infections play a significant role in pediatric asthma, infection alone does not equal asthma. Studies that evaluate the combination of genetic, immunologic, and environmental factors, including the role of infections, will ultimately lead to the best ways to control and prevent asthma.

References

1. Hahn DL, Dodge RW, Golubjatnikov R. Association of *Chlamydia pneumoniae* (strain TWAR) infection with wheezing, asthmatic bronchitis, and adult-onset asthma. *JAMA*. 1991;266:225-230.
2. Johnston SL, Martin RJ. *Chlamydophila pneumoniae* and *Mycoplasma pneumonia*: a role in asthma pathogenesis? *Am J Respir Crit Care Med*. 2005;173:1078-1089.
3. Gern JE, Lemanske RF. Infectious triggers of pediatric asthma. *Ped Clin North Am*. 2003;50:555-575.
4. Martin RJ. Infections and asthma. *Clin Chest Med*. 2006;27:87-98.
5. Richeldi L, Ferrara G, Fabbri LM, Lasserson TJ, Gibson PG. Macrolides for chronic asthma. *Cochrane Database Sys Rev*. 2005;19:CD002997.

WHAT DO PATIENTS WITH ASTHMA NEED TO KNOW ABOUT ENVIRONMENTAL CONTROL, AND WHAT IS THE EVIDENCE TO SUPPORT THESE INSTRUCTIONS?

Stephen J. McGeady, MD

Environmental control is a vast topic, and an in-depth review is beyond the scope of this chapter. The reader is referred to several excellent reviews if additional information is desired.[1-3] The asthmatic patient's environment includes both the indoors and the outdoors, and potential offending agents may be pollutants that aggravate asthma by their irritant or pro-inflammatory properties or allergens that cause asthma by causing an allergic airway reaction. Some pollutants may also skew immune responses to newly encountered antigens toward allergic responses, thereby expanding the number of potentially offending allergens. The various environmental factors of concern will be considered by primary location and recommended remedies described.

Outdoor pollutants include a large number of compounds, such as sulfur dioxide, nitric oxide, various volatile organic compounds and their metabolites and ozone. There are also particulate materials that may be harmful to asthmatic subjects, and these include diesel exhaust particles from motor vehicles and the particulate effluents of coal and power plants. Although the mechanism is not well-understood, ozone and diesel exhaust particles are able to produce an enhanced allergic response when individuals are exposed to an allergen to which they are sensitive.[4] Diesel exhaust particles have also been reported to skew immune responses to newly encountered antigens toward allergy.[1] The accumulated evidence that air pollutants encountered outside of the home are harmful to asthmatics is overwhelming, and there is convincing evidence that avoidance of these pollutants can have beneficial effects on asthma.[5]

Prevention of exposure to these asthma-aggravating pollutants, however, relies almost exclusively on avoidance, and that often includes either remaining indoors while pollutant levels are high or a change of residence out of an area where the pollutant is found. Relocation may not be realistic for some, especially those in lower socioeconomic strata, and this reality may account for part of the poor asthma outcomes seen in impoverished patients. The benefits of avoidance of high levels of air pollution have been documented in several reports. In one such report, the prevalence of respiratory illness in a town in Utah decreased during a strike that closed a steel mill for 1 year. While the mill was inactive, both the level of aerosolized particulates and the prevalence of respiratory disease, including asthma, decreased markedly. When the strike was settled and the mill resumed operation, both particulate levels in the atmosphere and respiratory disease in the community returned to pre-strike levels.[5] A similar observation was made when the city of Atlanta decreased motor vehicle traffic during the 1996 Olympics in an attempt to decrease summer ozone. Both the ozone level and asthma morbidity were reduced for the duration of the games.[6]

Outdoor allergens of concern include all of the aero-allergens that cause increases in asthmatic symptoms by eliciting allergic inflammation. These include primarily pollen and mold allergens, which occur on a seasonal basis. As noted in the earlier discussion of allergic asthma triggers (see Question 5), demonstrating a direct cause-and-effect relationship between these allergens and increased asthma symptoms has been difficult. In some allergic patients, however, there does appear to be a tendency for asthma symptoms to flare up at times when specific aero-allergens are at high levels. It is also a very common complaint that a child's asthma attacks are precipitated by "weather changes," and while weather changes involve a series of complicated atmospheric alterations, they may involve increased pollen and mold spore counts as these allergens are pushed ahead of advancing weather fronts. *Alternaria* mold spores in particular have been reported to be a risk factor for respiratory arrest and for death in children and young adults with asthma in the summer and early fall.[8]

Avoiding outdoor allergens is difficult but can sometimes be achieved by simply remaining indoors. This level of confinement is often impractical, and the negative effect on a child's psychosocial development and self-esteem should be a consideration before undertaking it. If outdoor exposure is unavoidable or deemed appropriate, it is sometimes possible to control the asthma symptoms with medications. Consideration can also be given to allergen immunotherapy, which may modulate symptoms if an outdoor allergen exposure is the apparent cause of asthma.

Indoor pollutants that may aggravate asthma include environmental tobacco smoke (ETS), which has been associated with several pathologic respiratory conditions and has been clearly connected to asthma exacerbations.[9,10] ETS contains a toxic mixture of irritant gases and particulates that are laced with polyaromatic hydrocarbons, which have the potential to generate oxidant species that inflame airway mucosa.[1] These compounds also skew immune responses to newly encountered antigens toward allergic responses. The burning of other biomass, such as in fireplaces, may produce a similar array of aerosolized compounds to ETS, although the concentration of these pollutants is almost always lower than that observed in ETS exposure. In addition to the byproducts of biomass incineration, nitrogen dioxide (NO_2) is a significant indoor pollutants. The origin of which is usually natural gas-burning appliances, especially when these are poorly maintained or inadequately ventilated. NO_2 is a known precursor to ozone in the outdoors, but, indoors, it acts by itself as a promoter of airway inflammation and is well-known to be associated with increased asthma symptoms.[11,12] The presence of biologically derived agents, such as endotoxin, has been associated with increased airway inflammation. These compounds are associated with the numbers of animals, including dogs, cats, and humans residing in a given home. The presence of endotoxin from gram-negative bacteria, 1-3 β glucans from molds, and products derived from gram-positive bacteria can cause airway inflammation directly, but may also influence the immune response to potential allergens toward allergic inflammation.[13]

Intervention to achieve avoidance of indoor pollutants primarily consists of the remediation steps that are obvious. ETS avoidance can best be achieved by discontinuing tobacco smoking altogether or at least confining it to the outdoors. The aerosolized products of wood or other biomass burning can be minimized by ensuring that the fireplace chimney is functioning optimally. NO_2 levels can be decreased when natural gas-burning appliances are made to function efficiently and are properly ventilated. Because endotoxin and biologically derived products seem to increase in direct proportion to the number of animals and humans in the home, keeping these inhabitant numbers to a reasonable level that is consistent with the size of the home offers one means of control, while another is maintaining a measure of cleanliness sufficient to prevent accumulation of these potentially harmful compounds.

Indoor allergens that may aggravate asthma include some that are highly airborne, while others are heavier and tend to settle. The best characterized of these heavy allergens are the house dust mites (HDMs). HDMs are found in fabric and bedding in their greatest numbers, and it is the droppings of the HDMs that are the principal source of allergens. The allergenic particles of HDM are heavy, and while they may be briefly aerosolized by dusting or vacuuming, they settle soon after. The greatest exposure to HDM allergen takes place while in bed because HDM are present in largest numbers in bedding, and a considerable fraction of a person's day is spent sleeping. In contrast to HDM allergen, the allergenic particles from cats and dogs are highly airborne and remain suspended for many hours. The property of remaining airborne together with the inherent allergenicity of dog and cat emanations makes these allergens readily inhaled and a major provoking stimulus in many asthmatic children. The allergens of rodents, which may be present in homes either as vermin or as pets, are not as well studied as are dog and cat, but data from occupational exposures and from the National Cooperative Inner Cities Asthma Study clearly illustrates the potential for rodent allergens to cause or aggravate asthma.[14] This same study of asthma in the inner cities has implicated cockroach allergy as being associated with asthma as well.[15] Like HDM allergen, cockroach allergen is a weighty particle and is aerosolized primarily during vacuum cleaning of a home infested by these insects. Mold spores are found in all environments both indoor and outdoor, but thrive in the presence of humidity. Thus, homes that have water damage, especially if the water is persistent, will have growing mold colonies and large numbers of airborne mold spores. As noted for outdoor molds, these spores can aggravate asthmatic symptoms.

Intervention to reduce indoor allergen exposure will vary with the specific allergen. As noted, HDM and cockroach allergens are weighty, and, consequently, air filtration with high-efficiency particulate air (HEPA) filters is not effective. Instead, it is recommended that mattresses and pillows be covered with impenetrable covers and bedding be washed at 7- to 14-day intervals in 130°F water. Vacuuming should be done with a double-thickness vacuum collection bag or HEPA filter.[14] In attempting to minimize allergen exposure to domestic pets, removal of the animal from the home is best, but seldom acceptable. HEPA air cleaners are helpful in reducing pet allergen exposure due to the aerodynamic properties of these animals' allergens. More important, however, is the removal, where possible, of reservoirs of allergen such as sofas and carpeting. Last, washing the pet on a frequent basis (eg, weekly) has been shown to diminish the allergen shedding.[16] For rodents and cockroaches, the obvious solution is to eliminate the infestation through eradication procedures. Mold remediation can be accomplished with any number of commercially available fungicides, but unless the source of moisture is eliminated, the mold will re-appear.

While published reviews of single interventions in control of indoor allergens have sometimes cast them as ineffective, the more carefully conducted studies have shown efficacy, particularly for HDM control. When a comprehensive approach to improving indoor air quality is carried out, the evidence is that there is a decrease in asthma symptoms and severity.[17]

References

1. Peden DB. Air pollution: indoor and outdoor. In: Adkinson NF, Bochner BS, Busse NW, Holgate SF, Laranske JR, Simons FER, eds. *Middleton's Allergy Principles and Practice.* 7th ed. St. Louis, MO: Mosby Elsevier. 2009: 495-508.
2. Platts-Mills TAE. Indoor allergens. In: Adkinson NF, Bochner BS, Busse NW, Holgate SF, Laranske JR, Simons FER, eds. *Middleton's Allergy Principles and Practice.* 7th ed. St. Louis, MO: Mosby Elsevier. 2009:539-556.
3. Custovic A. Allergen control in the prevention and management of allergic disease. In: Adkinson NF, Bochner BS, Busse NW, Holgate SF, Laranske JR, Simons FER, eds. *Middleton's Allergy Principles and Practice.* 7th ed. St. Louis, MO: Mosby Elsevier. 2009:1447-1458.
4. Peden DB. The epidemiology and genetics of asthma risk associated with air pollution. *J Allergy Clin Immunol.* 2005;115:213-219.
5. Pope CA 3rd. Respiratory disease associated with community air pollution and a steel mill, Utah Valley. *Am J Public Health.* 1989;79:623-628.
6. Friedman MS, Powell KE, Hutwagner L, Graham LM, Teague WG. Impact of changes in transportation and commuting behaviors during the 1996 Summer Olympic Games in Atlanta on air quality and childhood asthma. *JAMA.* 2001;285:897-905.
7. Denning DW, O'Driscoll BR, Hogaboam CM, Bowyer P, Niven RM. The link between fungi and severe asthma: a summary of the evidence. *Eur Respir J.* 2006;27:615-626.
8. O'Hollaren MT, Yunginger JW, Offord KP, et al. Exposure to an aeroallergen as a possible precipitating factor in respiratory arrest in young patients with asthma. *N Engl J Med.* 1991;324:359-363.
9. Gergen PJ. Environmental tobacco smoke as a risk factor for respiratory disease in children. *Respir Physiol.* 2001;28:39-46.
10. Gold DR. Environmental tobacco smoke, indoor allergens, and childhood asthma. *Environ Health Perspect.* 2000;(108 Suppl 4):643-651.
11. Brunekrsef B, Houthuijs D, Dykstra L, et al. Indoor nitrogen dioxide exposure and children's pulmonary function. *J Air Waste Management Assoc.* 1990;40:1252-1256.
12. Neas LM, Dockery DW, Ware JH, Spengler JD, Speizer FE, Ferris BJ Jr. Association of indoor nitrogen dioxide with respiratory symptoms and pulmonary function in children. *Am J Epidemiol.* 1991;134:204-219.
13. Virchow JC Jr, Julius P, Matthys H, Kroegel C, Luttmann W. CD14 expression and soluble CD14 after segmental allergen provocation in atopic asthma. *Eur Respir J.* 1998;11:317-323.
14. Matsui EC, Simons E, Rand C, et al. Airborne mouse allergen in the homes of inner-city children with asthma. *J Allergy Clin Immunol.* 2005;115:358-363.
15. Rosenstreich DL, Eggleston P, Kattan M, et al. The role of cockroach allergy and exposure to cockroach allergen in causing morbidity among inner-city children with asthma. *N Engl J Med.* 1997;336:1356-1363.
16. Platts-Mills TA, Vaughan JW, Carter MC, Woodfolk JA. The role of intervention in established allergy: avoidance of indoor allergens in the treatment of chronic allergic disease. *J Allergy Clin Immunol.* 2000;106: 787-904.
17. Morgan WJ, Crain EF, Gruchalla RS, et al. Inner-city Asthma Study Group. *N Engl J Med.* 2004;351:1068-1080.

SECTION V

ASTHMA OUTPATIENT

How Is Asthma Diagnosed
in Infancy and Childhood?

Alia Bazzy-Asaad, MD

Asthma is the most common chronic respiratory disease of childhood. Recent statistics show that 6.7 million or 9.1% of children in the United States have asthma,[1] accounting for 12.8 million absences from school each year. It is the third most common cause of hospitalization for children younger than 15 years and has been associated with a greater likelihood of preventable hospitalization in people with other diseases, such as diabetes.[2] Asthma disproportionately affects minority children. Non-Hispanic Black children are most likely to have either been diagnosed with asthma or still have asthma (20% and 15%), followed by Hispanic children (13% and 9%), and non-Hispanic White children (11% and 7%). Also, children in impoverished families are more likely to have been diagnosed with asthma or to still have asthma (17% and 12%) than children in families that were not impoverished (12% and 8%).[1] Among Hispanics, Puerto Rican children have the highest prevalence of lifetime asthma (26%) and recent asthma attacks (12%) compared with non-Hispanic Black children (16% and 7%, respectively), non-Hispanic White children (13% and 6%, respectively), and Mexican children (10% and 4%, respectively).

One suspects the diagnosis of asthma when an individual presents with recurrent coughing or wheezing episodes. However, it is well-known that not all cough or wheezing is indicative of asthma, as many other conditions may present with these symptoms. So, to establish the diagnosis of asthma, current guidelines recommend that one demonstrate that a patient has 1) episodic symptoms, 2) symptoms that are reversible, and 3) no other diagnosis that would explain the symptoms.[3] Fulfilling these criteria may not be easy in infants and young children, making the diagnosis of asthma challenging in this age group. In general, confirming the first component, the presence of episodic symptoms, can be accomplished at almost any age by obtaining a detailed medical history. The level of detail is quite extensive and is described in the National Asthma Education and Prevention Program *Expert Panel Report 3*.[3] Some of the important elements of the history include the type of symptoms (cough, wheeze, dyspnea, chest tightness, and sputum production), factors that trigger the symptoms (viral respiratory illness, environmental allergens or irritants, tobacco smoke, emotions, and exercise), pattern and seasonality of symptoms, past medical history, family history, and the presence of other conditions, such as gastroesophageal reflux or sinus disease. Combining the information obtained from the history with a thorough physical examination is the important next step. The physical exam should not focus on the lung exam exclusively. This is because, unless the child is acutely ill, the chest and lung exam may be perfectly normal. Therefore, the search for clues begins with a "head to toe" exam to find signs that indicate an allergic predilection (evidence of rhinitis or eczema), the presence of confounding factors such as gastroesophageal reflux (eg, hoarse voice), or the possibility of a diagnosis other than asthma, such as the presence of digital clubbing. The latter should not be present in a patient with asthma.

Confirming reversibility of symptoms is usually accomplished in 2 ways: clinical history and pulmonary function testing. The commonly recommended pulmonary function test is spirometry, which measures exhaled volumes and flows during a forced expiratory maneuver. This maneuver requires cooperation of the subject and the ability to follow instructions. The data generated are then compared to reference or "predicted" values from healthy subjects with the same anthropometric characteristics (age, gender, height, and race/ethnicity).[4] To demonstrate the presence of reversible airflow obstruction, the maneuver is performed before and following administration of a bronchodilator. Spirometry can be easily performed in the office setting in older children and adults. Because infants and young children cannot cooperate and follow commands, specialized equipment is required that is not readily available outside of specialized medical centers. In our experience, it is generally possible to obtain reliable data using standard spirometry equipment and the appropriate reference value starting at between 5 and 6 years of age.

Because most children develop asthma before the age of 5 years, making the diagnosis in infancy and early childhood is important to ensure proper treatment of underlying inflammation and symptoms. If a child presents with episodic symptoms and has a physical exam that is either within normal or suggests atopy, a therapeutic trial of asthma medications would be a reasonable approach to confirming the diagnosis. This is because a child with a different underlying condition (eg, cystic fibrosis or ciliary dyskinesia) would not be expected to improve significantly without adding other therapies, such as airway clearance or antibiotics.

A second factor that complicates the diagnosis of asthma in infants and young children is the finding that there are several wheezing phenotypes in this age group.[5] The phenotypes that have been identified in young children include transient early wheezers who have symptoms starting in infancy and resolving by age 3 to 5 years; non-atopic wheezers whose symptoms also start in infancy and are triggered by lower respiratory viral illness. In this group, symptoms persist during the first decade and are not associated with allergic sensitization. The third phenotype is the atopic wheezing persistent asthma phenotype. These children will have symptoms before age 6 years and have evidence of allergic sensitization and increased airway hyper-responsiveness. They are also at risk for loss of lung function, and hence early intervention with the appropriate asthma therapies may be key to preventing the loss of lung function, although definitive evidence to support this notion continues to be lacking. Using data collected from the Tucson Children's Respiratory

Study, a longitudinal study of respiratory illness in children, Castro-Rodriguez and colleagues were able to identify factors that increased a child's risk of developing chronic asthma.[6] The factors include frequent wheezing in infancy up to age 3 years and either 1 of 2 major risk factors (parental history of asthma or eczema) or 2 of 3 minor risk factors (eosinophilia, wheezing without colds, and allergic rhinitis). This index, now termed the Asthma Predictive Index (API), has a positive predictive value of 59% if the child has only one wheezing episode by age 3 years and 76% if the child has frequent wheezing by age 3 years. This index is therefore a useful tool when one is trying to determine the wheezing phenotype in a child age 3 years and younger. It has also been used in many recent wheezing/asthma research studies of infants and young children where the goal was to recruit children who are at increased risk for developing chronic asthma.

Summary

Diagnosing asthma in infants and young children poses challenges that are based primarily on the lack of easily obtainable pulmonary function measures. However, the risk of developing chronic asthma can be reasonably predicted using information that is easily obtained from a detailed medical history. In addition, response to asthma therapy provides another method of confirming the diagnosis in many cases.

References

1. Bloom B, Cohen RA, Freeman G. Summary health statistics for U.S. children: National Health Interview Survey, 2008. *Vital Health Stat 10.* 2009;244:1-81.
2. Niefeld MR, Braunstein JB, Wu AW, Saudek CD, Weller WE, Anderson GF. Preventable hospitalization among elderly Medicare beneficiaries with type 2 diabetes. *Diabetes Care.* 2003;26:1344-1349.
3. National Asthma Education and Prevention Program. *Expert panel report 3 (EPR-3): guidelines for the diagnosis and management of asthma.* Bethesda, MD: National Heart, Lung, and Blood Institute, 2007. NIH publication no. 08-4051.
4. Pellegrino R, Viegi G, Brusasco V, et al. Interpretative strategies for lung function tests. *Eur Respir J.* 2005;26:948-968.
5. Stein RT, Martinez FD. Asthma phenotypes in childhood: lessons from an epidemiological approach. *Paediatr Respir Rev.* 2004;5:155-161.
6. Castro-Rodriguez JA, Holberg CJ, Wright AL, Martinez FD. A clinical index to define risk of asthma in young children with recurrent wheezing. *Am J Respir Crit Care Med.* 2000;162(4 Pt 1):1403-1406.

I AM A BUSY PEDIATRICIAN. HOW CAN I INTEGRATE EFFECTIVE ASTHMA MANAGEMENT INTO MY PRACTICE?

Amy Renwick, MD

As a common pediatric problem with established national guidelines, asthma is well-suited to a standardized approach to outpatient management. Many tools for asthma management exist and are readily available, though you may want to adapt them for your practice. Some good sources for asthma materials include the National Heart, Lung, and Blood Institute (NHLBI) summary report, the American Lung Association, KidsHealth. org, and HealthyChildren.org.

The first step is to flag the charts (whether paper or electronic) of children with asthma, so they can be easily identified at office visits and for outreach efforts, such as influenza vaccination and tobacco prevention reminders. Set up your charts to make it easy to track the frequency and severity of exacerbations, including those requiring an emergency department visit, helping you decide when to step therapy up or down. Some offices also flag charts of severe asthmatics and have separate triage mechanisms and treatment algorithms for these at-risk patients. An asthma action plan, which serves as a summary of the patient's triggers and medication regimen, should also be readily available in the chart.

If patients may be seen by different providers within a group, agree amongst yourselves on a standard approach to education, use of controller medications, exacerbation management, etc. Patients will get a single, clear message, and providers will save time when covering each other's patients. Have your group's plan and general guidelines posted in charts or exam rooms for reference. This is not to imply a "cookie-cutter" or "one size fits all" management paradigm, but rather should ensure and optimize the adoption of well-established and published best practices. The overall goals of asthma management are fairly straightforward and uniform, and therefore it is often possible to align the practices of several providers to attain these outcomes (Table 21-1).

Schedule routine asthma follow-up visits separate from health maintenance visits, especially for children who have moderate to severe asthma. The NHLBI guidelines

Table 21-1

Goals of Guideline-Based Asthma Management

Reduce Impairment	Reduce Risk

• Minimize or prevent chronic symptoms
• Normalize sleep and activity levels
• Minimize use of rescue medication for breakthrough symptoms
    ○ Twice a week during the day
    ○ Twice a month during the night
• Maintain normal or near-normal lung function
• Obtain parental partnership and satisfaction with care
	• Prevent exacerbations
	• Prevent emergency room visits and hospitalizations
	• Prevent loss of lung function
	• Prevent reduced lung growth
	• Prevent adverse effects of therapy

recommend tailoring the interval between asthma visits to the severity and stability of each patient's condition, with a visit suggested at least every 1 to 6 months. These dedicated appointments allow you and the family to focus solely on asthma. Use the time to assess triggers, degree of control, and barriers to control; agree on treatment goals; discuss the care plan and make adjustments when indicated; and provide education and resources for home management. You may want to arrange for either an asthma visit or the annual physical to occur in the autumn to ensure that these high-risk children get influenza vaccine early in the season.

During the routine asthma follow-up visit, it is important to touch on the four key elements of asthma management. These include 1) assessment of control and symptom monitoring, including the assessment of lung function if possible, 2) patient education, 3) environmental control and assessment of co-morbid medical conditions, and 4) medical management, including drug delivery systems. By touching on each of these components at every office visit for asthma, a complete assessment will be ensured, medical red flags and knowledge gaps will be uncovered, and asthma outcomes will be enhanced. Tools can be developed to provide structure to a visit, and, with enough practice and clinical experience, touching on each of these aspects of asthma management, tools tailored to the needs of an individual patient will become second nature. A general structure for an asthma visit is presented in Table 21-2.

There is no single strategy for assessing asthma control and/or risk, but many different questionnaires are available to make this process more streamlined and standardized (Table 21-3). An example of these is the Asthma Control Test (ACT), which is widely available, is easy for parents and kids to use, and has been validated as a clinical assessment tool. Similarly, you can develop your own tool or prompt for tracking symptom severity. Whatever is decided, be certain to collect history related to triggers, symptom control, quality of life, and medications. Most questionnaires can be filled out in advance of the visit or while the patient is waiting to be seen. Choose a format that allows for quick review of the answers, particularly the most pertinent positives and negatives. Focusing

Table 21-2

Key Components of an Asthma Follow-Up Visit

1. *Overall Patient Assessment and Clinical Monitoring*	Severity related
	• Symptom scores
	  o Detailed history
	  o Assessment tool
	Risk related
	• Exacerbations
	  o Mild asthma flares
	  o Flares requiring oral steroids
	  o Unscheduled office visits
	  o Emergency department visits
	  o Hospitalizations
		Clinical monitoring
		• Objective measures of lung function
		  o Spirometry (preferred)
		  o Peak flow monitoring
			Physical examination
			• Features that suggest asthma
			  o Atopic features
			• Features that suggest an alternative diagnosis
			  o Failure to thrive
			  o Nasal polyposis
			  o Severe hyperinflation
			  o Crackles on auscultation
			  o Digital clubbing

2. *Patient Education*	• Targeted to the needs of the patient	• Three "Ds"
		  o Drugs to treat asthma
		  o Delivery systems for medications
		  o Devices for clinical monitoring
			• Other topics as indicated

3. *Environmental Review and Medical Comorbidities*	• Allergic triggers
	• Irritants (especially tobacco smoke)
		• Other triggers
		  o Exercise
		  o Respiratory viruses
			• Review of comorbid conditions
			  o Existing conditions controlled
			  o New condition apparent
			  o Review of testing results
			  o Additional testing required

4. *Medical Management*	• Does assessment of risk/control suggest any changes?	• Review and update asthma action plan	• Medication adherence • Side effects of medications

---

Table 21-3

Asthma Assessment Instruments

- Asthma Control Test (ACT)
  - 5 items
  - http://www.asthmacontrol.com
- Asthma Therapy Assessment Questionnaire (ATAQ)
  - 3 items
  - http://www.asthmacontrolcheck.com
- Asthma Control Questionnaire
  - 6 items
  - http://www.qoltech.co.uk/acq.html

---

on the recent time interval, 2 to 4 weeks, for symptom quantification reduces the risk of recall inaccuracies, which become more common as children and families reach further back into their memory banks to answer questions. Some tools are designed specifically for child self-report.

Older children—starting at age 6 or 7 years—should be queried in addition to the parents, as there may be significant differences between parent and child descriptions of symptoms and medication use. In most studies, the children themselves reported higher levels of symptoms than their parent or adult caregiver. This is not surprising because parents may not be aware of symptoms that occur on the playground, in the classroom, or in the middle of the night. So, it is critical to ask! Forms can also give teens and preteens an opportunity to disclose privately whether they smoke or are exposed to smoke when they are with friends. For example, there is a child-friendly version of the ACT that can be completed by school-aged children and is validated for use in children aged 4 to 11 years.

Education, an important component of all asthma visits, doesn't all have to be done by the physician. Take advantage of materials, such as videos and handouts, to cover key asthma topics. Train nurses or other office staff to review techniques for the proper use of peak flow meters, nebulizers, and inhalers with patients and parents. Selected "hot topics" in asthma education are listed in Table 21-4 and are discussed in detail in later chapters. Obviously, this list is not comprehensive but serves as a jumping-off point. Education must be relevant to the needs of the individual patient. It may even be practical to have one of the office staff become certified as an asthma educator if the patient volume and practitioner interest are high enough.

A written asthma action plan is the cornerstone of home asthma management. Used properly, it will guide families through appropriate use of routine medications and early recognition and treatment of exacerbations. This will reduce unnecessary calls and visits to your office and decrease the odds of a more severe exacerbation. Develop a paper or electronic template that can be quickly filled in with individual details. To be most effective, action plans should be concise, clearly presented, legible, and in language that is easily understood by caregivers.

Table 21-4
Key Knowledge Gaps to Address in Asthma Education

- Asthma action plan
- Peak flow monitoring
- Recognition of asthma flare
- Recognition of respiratory distress/emergency
- Response to increases in symptoms and attacks
- Environmental control measures

Periodically review your office practices, looking for ways to streamline asthma care. Identify wasted effort, such as collecting information you do not use, and points of delay. Office staff and families are valuable sources of insight—ask them what they find frustrating. Consider whether your outcomes match your clinical and logistical goals; if not, reorganize your approach.

Asthma management in the office, even a busy office, can be enjoyable, rewarding, and even profitable. Using available and validated resources for patient assessment and education and having a reasonably standardized approach and guideline-based action plan will optimize outpatient management and ensure the best possible outcomes for your patients.

References

1. Weinberger M. Pediatric asthma and related allergic and nonallergic diseases: patient-oriented evidence-based essentials that matter. *Pediatric Health.* 2008;2:631-650.
2. Halbert RJ, Tinkelman DG, Globe DR, Lin SL. Measuring asthma control is the first step to patient management: a literature review. *J Asthma.* 2009;46:659-664.
3. Liu AH, Zeiger R, Sorkness C, et al. Development and cross-sectional validation of the Childhood Asthma Control Test. *J Allergy Clin Immunol.* 2007;119:817-825.
4. Chidekel A, Marshall P. Acute asthma exacerbations roundtable. *J Asthma Allergy Educators.* 2010;1:71-74.

WHAT ARE THE MOST CURRENT ASTHMA GUIDELINES FROM THE NATIONAL INSTITUTES OF HEALTH AND WHAT DO I NEED TO KNOW ABOUT THEM?

Alia Bazzy-Asaad, MD

The National Institutes of Health (NIH) asthma guidelines were developed to "help health care professionals bridge the gap between current knowledge and practice" and to provide "a general approach to the diagnosis and management of asthma."[1] The previous version of the guidelines was published in 1997 (EPR-2 Guideline for short), with an update focused on specific questions in 2002. The most current version of the guidelines (EPR-3 Guideline), which was published in 2007, provides modifications and additions based on new information generated from asthma research during the past 10 years and was developed after an extensive review of the literature to date.

The EPR-3 Guideline highlights several areas that are major changes from the preceding version, which are summarized in Table 22-1. An important change is an emphasis on asthma control and clarification of the difference between classifying asthma severity and assessing asthma control. Although the EPR-2 Guideline stated that asthma severity should be classified before instituting asthma medications, the concept was not always apparent to practitioners. We witnessed many situations in our own clinic where a child would require multiple medications to control asthma symptoms, yet he or she would be classified at the end of the visit as having "mild intermittent asthma" because his or her symptoms were infrequent. This issue was even more apparent when we moved to an electronic medical record with computerized decision support because the computer would determine severity based on frequency of symptoms. Interestingly, corrections by providers were uncommon. The new clear separation between classifying severity versus control has greatly alleviated this problem.

Severity classification has been revised to eliminate the "mild intermittent" category and replace it with "intermittent" as a distinct group, maintaining mild, moderate, and severe classifications in the persistent group. This change makes sense because it is

Table 22-1

Highlights of Major Changes in *Expert Panel Report-3* Guidelines

- New focus on monitoring asthma control as a goal of therapy
  - ○ New focus on impairment and risk as the 2 key domains of severity and control, and multiple measures for assessment
  - ○ Modifications in the stepwise approach to managing asthma long term
  - ○ New emphasis on multifaceted approaches to patient education, environmental control factors, or comorbid conditions that affect asthma
- Modifications to treatment strategies for managing asthma exacerbations

Adapted from National Asthma Education and Prevention Program. Expert panel report 3 (EPR-3): guidelines for the diagnosis and management of asthma—summary report 2007. *J Allergy Clin Immunol.* 2007;120(5 Suppl):S94-S138.

well-known that children may have intermittent wheezing episodes that can be severe. Hence, labeling them as having mild intermittent asthma may result in under-treatment on an ongoing basis. As will be described next, this issue is further addressed by the introduction of new domains of assessment.

Two new domains of assessment, impairment, and risk have been added to the concepts of severity and control. Impairment refers to events that are occurring at the present time (eg, frequency of symptoms), while risk refers to events that may happen in the future, such as asthma exacerbations. Impairment provides an assessment of the frequency and intensity of symptoms, as well as the functional limitation associated with these symptoms. A standardized approach to assessing the impairment domain in asthma control is recommended via the use of a validated questionnaire, such as the Asthma Control Test. Risk, on the other hand, provides an estimate of the likelihood of asthma exacerbations, as well as of the progressive loss of lung function over time. The latter is a particularly important consideration for children, in whom preventing loss of lung function is a critical therapeutic goal. Impairment and risk domains represent different manifestations of asthma and may respond to treatment differently. For example, patients who have more ongoing symptoms (ie, more impairment but few acute exacerbations, or less risk) would require step up of controller therapy. On the other hand, patients who have minimal ongoing symptoms but suffer frequent acute exacerbations, as may occur after exposure to an allergen or a viral illness, may not benefit from stepping up controller therapy but rather from having oral corticosteroids on hand for emergency use to prevent escalation to a severe exacerbation. Hence, assessment of these domains is useful whether one is assessing the severity of asthma in a medication-naive patient or assessing how well asthma is controlled once therapy has been initiated.

Another important change is the approach to stepwise care and the addition of a new pediatric age group. While in the EPR-2 Guideline, children older than 5 years of age were included in the same stepwise treatment plan as adults, the EPR-3 Guideline now separates children younger than 12 years of age from adults. In addition, infants and preschoolers ages 0 to 4 years follow a treatment approach that differs from the 5- to 11-year-old school-age group. The rationale for this change is based on the recognition of different asthma phenotypes depending on age, as well as the strength of the evidence that supports the therapeutic approach in each age group. Preschool children present a particular challenge because many wheeze with viral illness but not at other times and do not go on to develop chronic asthma.[2] Because of this, many practitioners were reluctant to treat these children with daily controller therapy. The EPR-3 Guideline recommends controller therapy for these children based on assessment in the risk domain (frequent exacerbations) and a positive Asthma Predictive Index (API). The API identifies risk factors for development of chronic asthma based on the presence of recurrent episodes of wheezing plus one of two major criteria (physician-diagnosed eczema or parental asthma) or two of three minor criteria (physician-diagnosed rhinitis, wheezing without colds, or peripheral blood eosinophilia ≥4%).[3]

It is important to emphasize that, while for adults the strength of evidence for the various therapies used to control asthma is generally strong, the same is not true for pediatric patients, and many of the recommendations for treating preschool children are based on expert opinion. For example, while the data reported by the PEAK study (Preventing Early Asthma in Kids)[4] showed decreased frequency of asthma exacerbations in preschool children treated with fluticasone, only children with a positive API were included. Therefore, the effectiveness of daily controller therapy in preschoolers without a positive API is not clear, although many practitioners will use controllers in this age group irrespective of API.

The role of lung function measurement has been re-emphasized in the EPR-3 Guideline. Spirometry continues to be the primary method of assessing airflow; however, in contrast to the EPR-2 Guideline, where emphasis was placed on measurement of FEV1 (forced expiratory volume in 1 second), the ratio FEV1/FVC (forced vital capacity) has now been included in the assessment of impairment in school-age children, adolescents, and adults. FEV1 is often normal in children, irrespective of severity of asthma, and has been shown in adults to correlate with risk of exacerbation. FEV1/FVC represents the relationship of expiratory flow to lung capacity (ie, to the largest volume that a subject can exhale forcefully). Because of this, it is a better representative of impairment of lung function because a low ratio indicates that expiratory flow is decreased in relation to what a patient can eventually exhale. An analogy would be blowing out a given volume of air (representing FVC) through a large- versus a small-diameter tube. Much less air will be blown through the small tube in the first second as compared to blowing through the large tube, even though eventually all the volume will be expelled.

A new emphasis has been placed on using a multifaceted approach to patient education, as well as to the assessment of environmental factors and comorbid conditions that may affect asthma control. A key educational message clearly stated in the EPR-3 Guideline is "teach and reinforce at every opportunity." Practitioners are encouraged to review basic facts about asthma; to explain the roles of and differences between controller and quick-relief medications; and to review patient skills regarding inhaler technique, identification of triggers and methods of avoidance, self-monitoring, and self-management skills. This is not limited to scheduled office visits but is recommended to occur at encounters such as by the school nurse, the pharmacist dispensing the medications, and during urgent visits. Identification of triggers (eg, exercise and comorbidities, such as rhinosinusitis, obstructive sleep apnea, and stressors) will impact the patient's management plan because these conditions will require treatments in addition to asthma controllers and relievers. Proper management of these conditions may allow for stepping down of controller therapy and better asthma control.

Modifications have been made to medication recommendations. Instead of four steps for treatment, there are now 6 steps. This is to allow more flexibility in treatment options and separation of therapy escalations that were included in steps 3 and 4. In steps 2 and 3, nedocromil has been removed as a preferred controller option for preschoolers with mild persistent asthma, but kept as an alternative. Combination therapy of inhaled corticosteroids plus long-acting beta-adrenergic agonists (ICS/LABA) (eg, fluticasone/ salmeterol or budesonide/formoterol) is now included as a preferred option, along with increasing the dose of ICS from low to medium for patients with uncontrolled symptoms who are at step 4. The change in the recommendation is based on the growth of evidence showing that combination therapy is equivalent or at times superior to doubling the dose of ICS alone in terms of symptom control and decreasing exacerbations. Leukotriene receptor antagonist is recommended as an adjunctive therapy in school-age children and not as monotherapy, even for mild persistent asthma, because of recent data showing ICS to be superior to montelukast in controlling asthma in 6- to 17-year-old children.[5]

The anti-IgE antibody omalizumab has been added as adjunctive therapy for adults with uncontrolled severe persistent asthma but not for children younger than age 12 because it is not approved in this age group.

Finally, levalbuterol has been added as a recommended therapy for acute exacerbations, while doubling the dose of ICS for home management of exacerbations has been eliminated because of lack of evidence for effectiveness. Adjunctive treatment with magnesium sulfate or heliox may be considered in severe exacerbations unresponsive to initial treatment. Referral to follow-up care and patient education at discharge from acute care (emergency department or hospital) are also emphasized.

References

1. National Asthma Education and Prevention Program. Expert panel report 3 (EPR-3): guidelines for the diagnosis and management of asthma—summary report 2007. *J Allergy Clin Immunol.* 2007;120(5 Suppl):S94-S138.
2. Stein RT, Martinez FD. Asthma phenotypes in childhood: lessons from an epidemiological approach. *Paediatr Respir Rev.* 2004;5:155-161.
3. Castro-Rodriguez JA, Holberg CJ, Wright AL, Martinez FD. A clinical index to define risk of asthma in young children with recurrent wheezing. *Am J Respir Crit Care Med.* 2000;162(4 Pt 1):1403-1406.
4. Guilbert TW, Morgan WJ, Zeiger RS, et al. Long-term inhaled corticosteroids in preschool children at high risk for asthma. *N Engl J Med.* 2006;354:1985-1997.
5. Sorkness CA, Lemanske RF Jr, Mauger DT, et al. Long-term comparison of 3 controller regimens for mild-moderate persistent childhood asthma: the Pediatric Asthma Controller Trial. *J Allergy Clin Immunol.* 2007;119: 64-72.

WHAT IS AN ASTHMA ACTION PLAN AND HOW CAN ONE BE INDIVIDUALIZED FOR MY PATIENTS?

Aaron S. Chidekel, MD

An asthma action plan is a critical component of safe and high-quality asthma management. It represents a confluence of several important principles of guideline-based asthma care: clinical monitoring, medical management, and patient education. Every patient being seen for asthma should be given a written asthma action plan, but, unfortunately, studies have shown that many patients are not. The asthma action plan provides clear guidance to a patient or family about what should be done and when and for which level of symptoms or peak expiratory flow rates, and it provides the information to let them know who should be called for assistance and when it is time to call. In short, the asthma action plan is the written roadmap that guides a patient and family in the direction of safe and effective asthma self-management (Table 23-1). It is well worth the time in the office to craft one in writing for each asthma patient.

Written asthma action plans have been shown to be more effective than oral action plans, and this fact stresses the importance of putting onto paper or into an electronic medical record what it is that the patient needs to do to manage his or her own or his or her child's asthma. Written action plans allow for the earlier detection of asthma symptoms and flares and thereby allow for earlier intervention. This timely and appropriate intervention translates into reductions in unscheduled visits to the office and emergency department and more importantly into decreased frequencies of hospitalization and death. Other important outcomes that have been enhanced through the use of written asthma action plans include the reduction in night-time asthma symptoms and in days missed from work or school. It is implied that the asthma action plan is combined with education regarding its use and that understanding of the action plan is confirmed with the patient at the time of its inception. This dual process of education and formulation of an asthma action plan is a critical combination to promote self- or family-directed asthma management that is safe and efficacious.

Table 23-1

Important Components of an Asthma Action Plan

- How to assess asthma control
  - o Symptom scores
  - o Peak expiratory flow rate
- How to quantify symptom severity
  - o Symptom frequency or severity
  - o Peak expiratory flow zones
- How to maintain asthma control
  - o Which medications to take for control and relief
- How much medication to take
- How often to take medications
- When to seek assistance
  - o When to call the physician's office
  - o When to call for emergency assistance

Asthma action plans can be based on symptoms, peak expiratory flow rates, or both. While there remains some controversy as to which type of plan may be most efficacious, this distinction is less important from a practical perspective. My personal opinion is that all asthma actions plans need to have a symptom-based component. Symptoms such as the frequency and severity of coughing, wheezing, chest tightness, night-time awakenings, and decreased activity tolerance are all important to include. Then, if the patient is using a peak flow meter, it can be incorporated as well. If the patient in question is too young or is resistant to using a peak flow meter, then peak flow values are not included in the asthma action plan. Perhaps the only time that it is critical to include peak flow readings in an asthma action plan is in those patients who are poor perceivers of asthma symptoms. It is important to define these patients with poor perception of asthma symptoms because they are at increased risk of adverse asthma outcomes and, in this case, the ongoing and structured use of peak flow monitoring is important. In general, peak flow zones are created in an asthma action plan based upon a person's "personal best" peak expiratory flow rate. The green zone is defined as 80% to 100% of the personal best peak expiratory flow rate, the yellow zone is defined as 50% to 80% of the personal best peak expiratory flow rate, and the red zone is defined as 50% or less of the personal best peak expiratory flow rate. I usually start the action plan with the best peak expiratory flow rate obtained in the office and then have the patient use the peak flow meter for 1 to 2 weeks at home to further define his or her "real world" personal best and adjust the action plan accordingly.

As alluded to, most asthma action plans are modeled in zones using a "traffic light" analogy of green, yellow, and red zones to depict times of safety, caution, and danger (Table 23-2). This model is familiar to patients and parents and is easy to construct and envision. More important than the colors of the zones is the content that each zone contains. The components of an asthma action plan must communicate clearly, concisely, and efficiently how the patient should be feeling, what the peak flow reading should be,

Table 23-2

Cardinal Features of an Asthma Action Plan

- Green zone status
  - Well-controlled asthma
  - Minimal symptoms
  - Peak flow 80% to 100% of personal best
  - Medications for daily control provided
- Yellow zone status
  - Asthma control is slipping
  - Risk for flare-up is increasing
  - Symptoms are evident at a mild to moderate level
  - Peak flow 50% to 80% of personal best
  - Instructions for medical intervention provided
  - When to call physician noted
- Red zone status
  - Asthma is dangerously out of control
  - Flare-up is occurring
  - Severe symptoms are noted
  - Peak flow is less than 50% of personal best
  - Instructions for medical intervention provided
  - When to call physician or 911 noted

and what the patient should be doing in each of the zones of their action plan. If asthma control is slipping, it should be clear to the patient what actions to take and for how long to take them prior to calling for help. Medications and dosages should be documented for each zone, and the physician's and other emergency phone numbers should be clearly listed as well. Action plans should also describe acceptable duration of symptoms for each level of the plan. For example, it may be acceptable for the patient to wait a certain amount of time at one level of the plan, but not at another. Many asthma action plans are available to use, and they are available in different languages so that the action plan can be provided in a patient's native language. Specific action plan templates are available for children, daycare, schools, after exacerbations, and after exercise. Pick the resources that are most appropriate for your own practice, and implement them for your patients with asthma.

As part of ongoing asthma management, it is important to keep the action plan up to date. Asthma action plans should be reviewed with the patient and family at each follow-up visit and should be updated with new information reflecting changes in medications or other clinical parameters. Patient and family concerns with the action plan should be queried and addressed. This ongoing conversation helps to establish a partnership with the patient and facilitates effective 2-way communication. It also encourages adherence to therapy by investing the patient and family in the care process. In addition to keeping the action plan up-to-date, it is important that the action plan be a part of the patient's medical record either in paper or electronic form, and in addition to providing a copy to the patient, it is also necessary to provide copies of the action plan to schools, daycare centers, summer camps, or any other place where the child will be spending significant time.

Summary

A written asthma action plan should be a part of the ongoing management of any child with asthma, and this evidence-based statement is strongly rooted in the medical literature. Action plans can be based on symptoms, peak expiratory flow rates, or a combination of these clinical parameters and should be individualized to the unique circumstances of the patient who is in front of you. Action plans should be kept current and represent a living document that provides guidance about the management of this important chronic disease. The collaborative process of action plan development further enhances the relationship between the patient and provider and improves the self-management skills of the patient and family. The asthma action plan, by combining the ongoing assessment of control with the process of patient education and medical management, is truly a cornerstone of guideline-based asthma care.

Suggested Readings

Lougheed MD, Lemiere C, Dell SD, et al. Canadian Thoracic Society Asthma Management Continuum—2010 Consensus Summary for children six years of age and over, and adults. *Can Respir J.* 2010;17:15-24.

Morris KJ. *Asthma action plans: putting them to use.* Retrieved from www.medscape.org/viewarticle/739738 on May 16, 2011.

National Asthma Education and Prevention Program. *Expert panel report 3 (EPR-3): guidelines for the diagnosis and management of asthma.* Bethesda, MD: National Heart, Lung, and Blood Institute, 2007. NIH publication no. 08-4051.

Rank MA, Volcheck GW, Li JT, Patel AM, Lim KG. Formulating an effective and efficient written asthma action plan. *Mayo Clin Proc.* 2008;83:1263-1270.

Zemek RL, Bhogal SK, Ducharme FM. Systematic review of randomized controlled trial examining written action plans in children. *Arch Pediatr Adolesc Med.* 2008;162:157-163.

WHAT IS EXERCISE-INDUCED ASTHMA?

Brad Bley, DO, CSCS and Aaron S. Chidekel, MD

Exercise-induced bronchospasm (EIB) involves airway narrowing that occurs transiently during and after exercise. EIB can have a major impact on athletic performance and quality of life and contributes to the larger problem of "exercise intolerance" that is a frequent presenting complaint among pediatric patients. Exercise-related breathing complaints are common, even among elite athletes. It is estimated that as many as 50% of elite winter athletes may have exercise-induced asthma (EIA).[1] It has also been estimated that approximately 10% to 15% of otherwise healthy children will have isolated EIB. Exercise intolerance and EIB are common among individuals with atopy and chronic asthma. It is reported that between 50% and 90% of children with co-existing asthma and as many as 30% to 40% of people with allergic rhinitis will have symptoms of EIB.[2,3] Among patients with chronic asthma, however, activity limitation is an important indicator of inadequate asthma control and can have significant health consequences to an active, healthy lifestyle.

A physician may see many cases of dyspnea with exercise throughout the year, and dyspnea is a common symptom with a broad differential diagnosis (see Question 31, Table 31-1). Feelings of shortness of breath are normal with exercise, and, therefore, not all patients who have exercise-induced dyspnea (EID) require treatment with bronchodilators, inhaled steroids, or even any diagnostic studies.[4] In fact, many will require no medical treatment whatsoever.

When approaching a patient with exercise intolerance or symptoms that might suggest EIB or EIA, there are 3 potentially related clinical scenarios to differentiate. The first is the patient with isolated EIB who does not have co-existing asthma. This patient has symptoms limited to exercise and has no other chronic airway symptoms or triggers. It may be useful to think of this as isolated intermittent asthma with exercise or just isolated EIB. The distinction is somewhat semantic. The second and third scenarios are inter-related and involve patients with definitive co-existing asthma. Therefore, these patients have true EIA because exercise is one of their identifiable asthma triggers. The second scenario is a patient with intermittent asthma who does not require chronic controller therapy but who also has asthma triggers other than exercise. The third and final scenario involves patients with persistent asthma who use a controller medication(s) and have symptoms of EIA.

Differentiating between patients with chronic asthma and EIA and those with isolated EIB is important because the assessment, management, and follow-up of these children will vary considerably. Furthermore, among patients with significant asthma, exercise-related complaints are very common (as high as 50% to 90%),[5] and control of these exercise-induced symptoms is an important goal of asthma therapy. Exercise is good for all children, and among those with asthma, exercise has many benefits, including an improvement in respiratory symptoms and quality of life. Exercise decreases the need for asthma medications; however, those children with more severe asthma will be at higher risk of an asthma exacerbation due to exercise and need to be managed and followed accordingly. Despite these different clinical scenarios, there are some commonalities that are important. Exercise-induced symptoms will vary with the specific activity, the intensity of the exercise, the ambient temperature, and the specific exercise environment, and this creates opportunities for management strategies that will help children with asthma find healthy and safe physical activities that can be incorporated into an active lifestyle.

EIA is often diagnosed clinically based on reported symptoms similar to those noted in asthma.[6] These symptoms include cough, wheeze, chest tightness, and congestion that are worsened or brought on by exercise. Patients may report feeling out of shape or being unable to keep up with their peers in gym, recess, or organized sports. Symptoms of EIA typically occur within the first 10 to 15 minutes of exercise, peak 8 to 15 minutes after exercise, and resolve about an hour after completion, but these symptoms have also been reported to occur throughout exercise as well.[7,8] A careful history of symptoms including the timing of their onset and the physical examination are important in the evaluation of shortness of breath with exercise, but they are not very sensitive or specific for EIB or EIA.[6,9,10,4] EIB and EIA are promoted by exercise in cold, dry air and the presence of air pollutants, allergens, or irritants. In a patient with co-existing asthma, the likelihood of worsened EIA is increased with the presence of another trigger, such as a viral respiratory tract infection or days with high pollen counts or poor air quality. Confounding all of this is the fact that dyspnea is a subjective complaint, and its specificity for any given diagnosis is low.[11] The challenge for physicians, therefore, is identifying those individuals with asthma and differentiating them from those with another cause for exercise intolerance. This is discussed in greater detail in Question 31.

The pathophysiology of EIB has not been completely elucidated, but several factors are believed to be important in its occurrence. Briefly, during exercise, there are large increases in ventilation that lead to both increased volumes of air flow and increased air flow rates. This inspired air must be filtered and humidified prior to entering the lower airways, and the changes in ventilation with vigorous exercise overcome the ability of the nose and upper airway to moisten, filter, and warm inspired air. This can result in the drying and cooling of the airway mucosa and in the deposition of allergens and pollutants. This may then result in airway inflammation and changes in pulmonary vascular tone in a susceptible host. Inflammation can lead to bronchospasm by stimulating airway smooth muscle contraction and can cause airway edema and mucous production.

Changes in vaso-motor tone can lead to vascular engorgement with resultant airway narrowing as well. This inflammatory and vaso-motor response in the lung is thought to underlie EIB. Similarly, there may be direct airway epithelial injury due to the occurrence of very high airflow rates with vigorous exercise. This model of the pathophysiology of airway inflammation and narrowing in response to exercise has direct clinical relevance to the management of EIB and will also be discussed further in Question 31.

Air pollution worsens both asthma and EIB. The increases in ventilation that accompany normal exercise lead to increased exposure to toxic components of air pollution, such as ozone, sulfur and nitrogen oxides, and particulate matter. These in turn promote airway injury and inflammation and worsen pulmonary dysfunction. Indoor environments, such as pools with irritating chlorine and ice rinks where fossil fuel burning ice machines can create pollution, and outdoor urban environments are all implicated in contributing to exercise dysfunction. Children may have environment-specific exercise difficulties due to the presence of pollutants and irritants, and physicians should be aware of these factors. Long-term studies have linked the risk of developing asthma with high levels of exercise in polluted communities. In one study, the risk of developing asthma was directly related to the number of sports that children played outdoors in communities with high ozone levels.[12] As clinicians, awareness of the exercise environment and air quality are important parts of the management of children with EIA and/or bronchospasm.

Identifying patients with asthma and EIA is critical from a public health standpoint. The promotion of regular exercise and healthy lifestyles is vitally important, and persistent asthma with EIA and EIB should not stand in the way of successful athletic performance. EIA and EIB have been reported even among elite athletes, and up to 10% to 11% of Olympic athletes are reported to have these conditions.[13] That said, as with any form of asthma, the risk of the disease must be carefully managed as well. Among sudden sports-related deaths, asthma was reported to be the cause in approximately 1% of these events. However, among asthma-related deaths that occurred during sports, 80% of these occurred in youth younger than 21 years of age, and half of these deaths occurred among patients age 13 to 17 years. In this study by Becker and colleagues, it was found that, among asthma deaths associated with a sporting event or physical activity occurring during a 7-year review period, 57% of deaths were among elite or competitive athletes, and nearly 10% of deaths occurred in athletes with no known history of asthma. Among the 90% of known asthma cases, however, only 5% were using a controller medication.[14]

Summary

Both EIA and EIB are common in pediatric patients, and these children with underlying airway reactivity need to be differentiated from other children with many other causes of EID. The difficult task in correctly identifying patients with EIA is often related to the intermittent and reversible nature of the patient's symptoms, and an asymptomatic patient may not have any physical examination findings whatsoever and may have normal baseline lung function. Accurately diagnosing and managing exercise-related problems in patients with asthma will be discussed in more detail in Question 31. Recognizing that exercise is both an important asthma trigger as well as a potential confounder is critical to differentiate among those patients who need more aggressive asthma management and those who simply need encouragement or reassurance.

References

1. Storms WW. Exercise-induced asthma in athletes: current issues. *J Asthma*. 1995;32:245-257.
2. Makker AC, Holgate ST. Mechanisms of exercise-induced asthma. *Eur J Clin Invest*. 1995;24:571-585.
3. Kobayashi RH, Mellion MB. Exercise-induced asthma, anaphylaxis and urticaria. *Prim Care*. 1991;18:809-831.
4. Heinle R, Linton A, Chidekel AS. Exercise-induced vocal cord dysfunction presenting as asthma in pediatric patients: toxicity of inappropriate inhaled corticosteroids and the role of exercise laryngoscopy. *Pediatr Asthma Allergy Immunol*. 2003;16:215-224.
5. Makker AC, Holgate ST. Mechanisms of exercise-induced asthma. *Eur J Clin Invest*. 1995;24:571-585.
6. Abu-Hasan M, Tannous B, Weinberger M. Exercise-induced dyspnea in children and adolescents: if not asthma then what? *Ann Allergy Asthma Immunol*. 2005;94:366-371.
7. Tan RA, Spector SL. Exercise-induced asthma. *Sports Med*. 1998;25:1-6.
8. Wallace JM, Stein S, Au J. Special problems of the asthmatic patient. *Curr Opin Pulm Med*. 1997;3:72-79.
9. Seear M, Wensley D, West N. How accurate is the diagnosis of exercise induced asthma among Vancouver schoolchildren? *Arch Dis Child*. 2005;90:898-902.
10. Parsons JP, Mastronarde JG. Exercise-induced bronchoconstriction in athletes. *Chest*. 2005;128:3966-3974.
11. Weinberger M, Abu-Hasan M. Perceptions and pathophysiology of dyspnea and exercise intolerance. *Pediatr Clin North Am*. 2009;56:33-48.
12. McConnell R, Berhane K, Gilliland F, et al. Asthma in exercising children exposed to ozone: a cohort study. *Lancet*. 2002;359:386-391.
13. Voy RO. The US Olympic Committee experience with exercise-induced bronchospasm. *Med Sci Sports Exerc*. 1986;18:328-330.
14. Becker JM, Rogers J, Rossini G, Mirchandani H, D'Alonzo GE Jr. Asthma deaths during sports: report of a 7-year experience. *J Allergy Clin Immunol*. 2004;113:264-267.

Suggested Readings

Cava JR, Danduran MJ, Fedderly RT, Sayger PL. Exercise recommendations and risk factors for sudden cardiac death. *Pediatr Clin North Am*. 2004;51:1401-1420.

Turcotte H, Langdeau JB, Thibault G, Boulet LP. Prevalence of respiratory symptoms in an athlete population. *Respir Med*. 2003;97:955-963.

WHAT IS NOCTURNAL ASTHMA?

Holger Link, MD

Nocturnal asthma is clinically defined as the presence of wheezing, coughing, or shortness of breath during the normal sleeping hours. The nocturnal symptoms are a reflection of airway inflammation and airway hyper-responsiveness. Lung function measurement during the night in a patient with nocturnal asthma would show a greater than 15% decrease in lung function from baseline as measured by forced expiratory volume in the first second (FEV1). However, the utility of lung function measurement is limited due to technical and logistical difficulties in performing the test at night and due to the fact that the child would have to be at least 6 years of age. Nocturnal asthma is common, and children with more severe daytime asthma symptoms are also likely to have more frequent and more severe nocturnal symptoms. Some children, however, may have symptoms only during the night.

The diagnosis of nocturnal asthma is based on a thorough asthma history that includes a direct exploration of night-time symptoms and sleep quality. Nocturnal asthma may go unnoticed unless the parents and child are specifically asked about wheezing, coughing, and shortness of breath after bedtime. In addition, asthma guidelines emphasize the importance of quantifying night-time symptoms in differentiating intermittent from persistent asthma as well as in the assessment of ongoing asthma control.

The burden of nocturnal asthma to the child's health and the family as a whole can be significant and is not necessarily limited to the respiratory system. Consolidated and restful sleep is essential for normal daytime functioning. Asthma and its treatment have many effects on sleep (Table 25-1). The wheezing and coughing that are associated with nocturnal asthma often disrupt normal sleep patterns and impair sleep quality. Conversely, treatment of the wheezing and coughing during the night with albuterol (or other sympathomimetic medications) can have the side effects of insomnia and disrupted sleep, and systemic corticosteroids have similar adverse effects on sleep. Disrupted sleep

Table 25-1

Asthma and Sleep

Impact of Asthma on Sleep	Impact of Asthma Medications on Sleep	

• Insomnia
• Excessive daytime sleepiness
• Nocturnal asthma symptoms
• Nocturnal bronchospasm
• Sleep-related hypoxemia
	Bronchodilators
	  • Insomnia
	Corticosteroids
	  • Insomnia
	  • Nightmares
		Theophylline
		  • Sleep disruption
		  • Insomnia
		Anti-histamines
		  • Sedation
		  • Excessive sleepiness
		    ○ First-generation
		      agents > Second-
		      generation agents

can lead to impairment in cognitive function, behavior, and mood. In addition, nightly awakenings from asthma can result in missed school days and learning problems. Missed school days often translate into missed days at work for parents, which can pose a serious financial burden to the family.

Multiple factors can contribute to a worsening of asthma symptoms during the night. Lung function varies with the time of day and is typically highest in the mid-afternoon and lowest in the early morning hours. The airways in patients with nocturnal asthma show increased inflammation during the night when compared to the daytime. This may be related to the physiologic nadir of endogenous corticosteroid production that occurs during the early morning hours. Furthermore, the sleep environment may directly contribute to the nocturnal symptoms. For example, a child with a dust mite allergy could have a higher nocturnal exposure to the dust mite allergen from bedding.

Commonly used asthma drugs might not work as well during the night as they do during the daytime for several reasons. For example, albuterol receptors (beta-2 adrenergic receptors) decrease in density and are less responsive during the night in patients with nocturnal asthma. A dose of albuterol that would lead to significant improvement in airflow during the daytime would therefore not result in the same improvement when given during the night. Another example of the nocturnal variation of drug efficacy can be found in glucocorticoids. Glucocorticoids have potent anti-inflammatory effects and are typically the first-line therapy for asthma. Unfortunately, glucocorticoid binding to its receptor is decreased in the early morning hours in asthmatic patients, therefore potentially decreasing the anti-inflammatory effects of externally administered and endogenous corticosteroids.

The first step in treating a child with nocturnal asthma is to make an accurate diagnosis via a thorough history. Keep in mind that not all parents and patients will bring up concerns about nightly symptoms on their own. Therefore, direct questioning about night-time cough, wheeze, shortness of breath, and rescue medication use is strongly recommended.

The second step is to review the patient's adherence to currently prescribed asthma medications and proper inhaler technique. You might be surprised to find that the child does not use a spacer device, exhales into the spacer, uses an empty inhaler, or uses albuterol daily instead of the inhaled steroid.

The third step is a detailed environmental history that should include asking about the bed (dust mite-proof covers?), animals (furry or feathered) that sleep in the room, and dust exposure. Make sure to eliminate any potential triggers from the sleep environment. Allergy testing might be of value if you are concerned about dust mite allergy or an allergy to a family pet.

The fourth step is to ask about symptoms that are suggestive of comorbid conditions like gastroesophageal reflux disease (GERD) or obstructive sleep apnea (OSA). Suddenly waking up from sleep with gasping for air would be suggestive of a reflux episode and resulting laryngospasm. Make sure to ask for bedtime eating habits in the infant and toddler with nocturnal wheezing and coughing because a child who falls asleep nursing or drinking from the bottle is at increased risk for aspiration. A trial of an acid blocking medication is reasonable when a clinical suspicion for GERD exists. In order to be sure that GERD is not the main trigger for the nocturnal symptoms, you should treat with the optimal dose of an antacid medication before calling it a failed response.

Children with nocturnal asthma should be screened for the presence of sleep apnea, as sleep disruption from sleep apnea can potentiate the sleep-disturbing effect of nocturnal asthma. In addition, you should be aware that untreated sleep apnea might contribute to increased nocturnal asthma severity in some patients. A couple of simple questions will help you screen for sleep apnea: Does your child snore, or is he or she a noisy breather? Does your child's breathing look comfortable during sleep? It can be a bit tricky sometimes to distinguish the wheeze from a snore. You might ask the parents if it seems to be harder for the child to breathe in or out (OSA harder to breathe in, asthma usually harder to breathe out).

An overnight sleep study or polysomnogram (PSG; Figure 25-1) can be helpful in distinguishing between asthma-related symptoms and sleep apnea. Remember that children with obesity and enlarged tonsils are at particularly high risk for OSA. Simply stated, a PSG is the simultaneous recording of multiple physiological parameters relevant to sleep and breathing. Its purpose is the diagnosis of sleep-related breathing problems and the identification of other types of sleep disorders. Electroencephalogram (EEG), chin electromyogram (EMG), and electro-oculogram (EOG) are measured to differentiate wake from sleep and to allow for the assessment of sleep architecture. The EEG montage is not sufficient to diagnose seizures. Airflow is measured at the mouth and nose, which along with respiratory motion sensors on the chest and abdomen establish the presence of the 3 types of apnea: central, obstructive, or mixed. Gas exchange is measured with pulse oximetry for oxygenation. In children, measurement of ventilation, most often by end tidal carbon dioxide ($EtCO_2$) recording, is recommended to identify obstructive hypoventilation. Body position and electrocardiogram (ECG) are recorded, as is the presence of limb movements with anterior tibialis EMG. The study is performed overnight under the direct observation of a trained polysomnography technician. As with lung function testing, it is critical to ensure that the sleep laboratory has the ability and experience to test children. This is an expensive and time-consuming test!

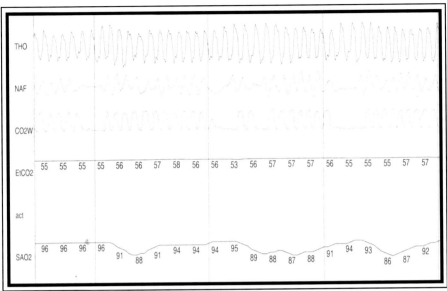

Figure 25-1. A series of respiratory tracings from a polysomnogram demonstrating obstructive apnea with oxyhemoglobin desaturation and hypercapnia. Thoracic impedance (THO) depicts chest movement or respiratory effort. Nasal airflow (NAF) represents airflow measured by nasal-oral thermistry. End-tidal carbon dioxide wave (CO2W) shows the flow measured by capnometry also at the nose. Oxygen saturation and end-tidal CO2 values are also depicted numerically. Obstructive apnea occurs when there is continued effort as shown by activity in the THO channel with absence of airflow in the NAF and CO2W channels. There are 4 episodes of obstructive apnea shown in this 2-minute epoch associated with oxyhemoglobin desaturations.

Once you are confident in your diagnosis, are comfortable that the patient is using the medications as prescribed with good technique, have taken a thorough environmental history, and have eliminated potential triggers and GERD or OSA as a contributing factor, you will likely need to step up the patient's asthma medications. You could also try delaying the dosing of the inhaled steroid to just before bedtime to provide better anti-inflammatory and symptom control in the early morning hours.

Summary

While isolated nocturnal asthma is uncommon, nocturnal asthma symptoms are both common and troublesome. Because asthma guidelines recommend specific assessment of nocturnal symptom frequency and severity, an evaluation of what happens after sleep onset and in the early morning hours is an important component of asthma management. Asthma and its therapy can have a major negative impact on sleep, and occasionally asthma and a primary sleep disorder co-exist. A systematic approach, as outlined above, can usually bring night-time symptoms under control either through the identification and treatment of an environmental trigger or a medical comorbidity or through enhanced education and medical management.

Suggested Readings

Alkhalil M, Schulman E, Getsy J. Obstructive aleep apnea syndrome and asthma: what are the links? *J Clin Sleep Med.* 2009;5:71-78.

Dean BB, Calimlim BC, Sacco P, Aguilar D, Maykut R, Tinkelman D. Uncontrolled asthma among children: impairment in social functioning and sleep. *J Asthma.* 2010:47:539-544.

Diette G. Nocturnal ashma in children affects school attendance, school performance, and parents' work attendance. *Arch Pediatr Adolesc Med.* 2000;154:923-928.

Ginsberg, D. An unidentified monster in the bed—assessing nocturnal asthma in children. *McGill J of Med.* 2009;12:31-38

Greenberg H, Cohen RI. Nocturnal asthma. *Curr Opin Pulm Med.* 2012;18:57-62

Hendeles L. Response to inhaled albuterol during nocturnal asthma. *J Allergy Clin Immunol.* 2004;113:1058-1062.

Sutherland E. Nocturnal asthma. *J Allergy Clin Immunol.* 2005;116:1179-1186

My Patient's Asthma Is Not Getting Better. What Treatment Options Do I Have?

Anita Bhandari, MD

It is difficult to know exactly how many patients have difficult-to-treat asthma because of the many terms that are used to describe these patients. Some commonly used terms include brittle asthma, steroid-dependent asthma, near fatal asthma, and refractory asthma. A recent review of uncontrolled asthma reported that approximately 20% of all asthmatics have severe asthma, of which 20% is inadequately controlled.[1] This group of patients deserves special attention because they are at a higher risk for adverse outcomes, including poor quality of life, multiple emergency department visits, and hospitalizations, and the individuals also are more likely to die from asthma.

Although there is no clear definition of refractory asthma in children, according to the American Thoracic Society, the definition of refractory asthma in adults requires that the patient must meet one or both major characteristics and 2 minor characteristics (as shown in Table 26-1) after adequate adherence and compliance with an asthma action plan and medications has been confirmed.[2] In children, as in adults, ensuring adequate adherence to and understanding of the medical management plan is critical and emphasized in the National Institutes of Health (NIH) guidelines. Similarly, reviewing potential environmental triggers and evaluating for the presence of comorbid conditions is critical. There are common comorbid states that may affect response to usual asthma medications, such as gastroesophageal reflux (GER), rhinitis, sinusitis, obstructive sleep apnea, obesity, and allergic bronchopulmonary aspergillosis. Because "all that wheezes is not asthma," particular attention should be paid to other conditions that may mimic asthma (Table 26-2) when patients are difficult to control with usual medications. These diagnoses should be ruled out before other asthma therapies are initiated.

When other medical conditions have been excluded and adequate compliance assured, the next step is to examine the patient's environment, which in a child, includes not only the home, but also places of day care and the school environment as well. Common

Table 26-1
Characteristics of Refractory Asthma

Major Characteristics	Minor Characteristics
1. Treatment with continuous or near-continuous use of oral steroids. 2. Requirement for treatment with high-dose inhaled corticosteroids (>50% of the time).	1. Requirement for daily treatment with controller medication in addition to inhaled corticosteroids. 2. Asthma symptoms requiring short-acting beta-agonist use on a daily or near-daily basis. 3. Persistent airway obstruction FEV1<80% predicted and diurnal variation of PEF>20%. 4. One or more urgent visits for asthma per year. 5. Three or more oral steroid bursts per year. 6. Prompt deterioration with 25% or less reduction in overall inhaled steroid dose. 7. Near fatal asthma event in the past.

Table 26-2
Common Causes of Cough and Wheeze in Children

Infant	Preschool Age	School Age
• GER • Cystic fibrosis • Congenital abnormalities of lung and airways (vascular rings/slings) • Tracheobronchomalacia • Ciliary dyskinesia • Congenital heart disease • Immunodeficiency • Bronchopulmonary dysplasia	• Cystic fibrosis • Ciliary dyskinesia • Foreign body inhalation • Aspiration • Immunodeficiency	• Cystic fibrosis • Ciliary dyskinesia • Immunodeficiency • Alpha-1 anti-trypsin deficiency • Vocal cord dysfunction • Malignancies

triggers of asthma, such as exposure to cigarette smoke, mold, rodents, roaches, and dust mites, can promote continued airway irritation and inflammation, which can be the cause for poor response to usual asthma medications. It is important to pose questions that explore the possibilities with parents and the child at each visit. Remembering to talk directly to the child is particularly important as all of us have occasionally been surprised and educated by their honest and relevant answers.

The first step in addressing severe or refractory asthma is to identify and adequately treat any asthma comorbidities. Then, adherence must be assured, and other medical conditions and environmental confounders must be considered and excluded. After this medical and psychosocial evaluation is completed, the next step is to maximize doses of usual asthma medications for severe asthma, including inhaled steroids, combination inhaled steroid and long-acting bronchodilator medications, and leukotriene inhibitors as per the National Heart, Lung, and Blood Institute (NHLBI) recommendations.[3] Patients with severe or refractory asthma usually require more than one controller medication (in addition to relief medications) and possibly even chronic oral corticosteroid therapy. A complete discussion of the use of chronic oral steroids is beyond the scope of this discussion, but a few factors should be kept in mind. The use of chronic oral steroids is reserved for those patients in whom standard therapy has been insufficient after thorough medical evaluation, environmental review, and asthma education. The dose of oral steroids is minimized using other controller medications, and whenever possible, the oral steroid is administered once daily or every other day to attempt to minimize steroid-related side effects. It is also assumed that any patient requiring this level of asthma therapy will also be followed by an asthma specialist, such as an allergist, pulmonologist, or both.

In addition to combinations or higher doses of standard asthma therapies, and the rare patient requiring chronic oral steroids, there are a few newer asthma medications on the horizon that may be used in addition to ones usually recommended. These are discussed further in the following paragraphs.

Additional therapy with newer agents such as omalizumab should be considered in patients with refractory asthma. Omalizumab is a humanized monoclonal antibody active against immunoglobulin-E (IgE) and is a treatment option in those patients who are not getting better with usual medications. This agent has been found to be especially useful in decreasing the number of acute exacerbations of asthma, emergency room visits, and hospitalizations in patients who are not well controlled even with higher doses of combination therapy.[4] The greatest benefit was seen in the patients with the lowest levels of lung function (FEV1). Omalizumab is administered as a subcutaneous injection every 2 to 3 weeks in the doctor's office. It is recommended that the patients be watched for 2 hours in the office after the dose for the first 3 doses because there is a risk of developing anaphylactic reaction with the risk being greatest for up to 2 hours after receiving the injection. After the patient has tolerated the first 3 doses well, the observation period can be decreased to 30 minutes for subsequent doses. A usual duration of 6 months is recommended to start with, and patients may stay on therapy longer if there is significant improvement in symptoms. The most feared side effect is anaphylaxis, which is unusual but may occur in 0.9% of the patients. There has been some concern about increasing rates of malignancy with this therapy as well; however, recent data do not support this concern. This is an expensive medication and costs about $500 to $2000 per month but is typically covered by most insurance carriers. I recommend that this therapy be initiated at the recommendation of a specialist (pulmonologist or an allergist) and the first 3 doses be given at the specialist's office, and from there on, visits can be alternated between the specialist's office and the primary care provider's (PCP) office. This strategy also is effective in maintaining a close level of collaborative follow-up. It is also my practice to obtain spirometry at least once every 4 weeks in patients who are on omalizumab.

Macrolide antibiotics are another therapy that is used in patients with refractory asthma. Macrolide antibiotics have been shown to decrease neutrophilic inflammation in patients with asthma, although a Cochrane review in 2005 concluded that there was insufficient evidence to recommend use of macrolides as add-on therapy for patients with severe asthma.[5] Recent studies have shown that clarithromycin when used in patients with severe non-eosinophilic asthma decreases inflammation and improves quality of life. In my practice, I have used macrolides (azithromycin) as add-on therapy in patients with difficult-to-treat asthma.

There are a couple of potential drugs presently in trials for treatment of severe asthma, including anti-IL-5 monoclonal antibodies, which have shown improvement in lung function (FEV1). Some of these have shown promise in clinical trials (SCH55700), while others (SB240563 and mepolizumab) have failed to show clinical benefit. Suplatast is an oral agent that blocks synthesis of cytokines; it has been tried and was found to be useful in children with food allergies and has been shown to decrease the incidence of asthma in this population. Further investigations are ongoing for patients with severe asthma. Other drugs with immunomodulatory effects, including methotrexate, cyclosporine, gold salts, troleandomycin, azathioprine, and chloroquine, have also been tried but have largely fallen out of favor because of their poor risk/benefit ratio.

A novel procedure called bronchial thermoplasty has recently been approved by the FDA for adult asthma patients. In patients with asthma, there often exists significant airway smooth muscle hypertrophy, which can be a result of airway remodeling from severe disease or as a result of chronic asthma therapies. Bronchial thermoplasty specifically targets airway smooth muscle. It involves a direct application of heat to the airway in an effort to decrease airway muscle mass. The procedure is usually done under sedation and typically lasts 30 minutes, similar to a flexible bronchoscopy. Usually, 3 such treatments are recommended. Five-year data in patients who received this therapy show marked improvements in quality of life, decreases in emergency room visits, increases in symptom-free days, decreases in bronchodilator use, decreases in severe asthma exacerbations, and decreases in work and school absences. There has been some concern regarding increased risk of developing side effects, such as an acute exacerbation of asthma requiring hospitalization following this procedure in patients with severe asthma.[6] At the present time, bronchial thermoplasty is not approved for use in children.

Summary

Refractory asthma is a high-risk and difficult situation. In those patients whose asthma is poorly responsive to standard therapy or who require multiple medications, I recommend that they be evaluated by an asthma specialist, such as an allergist, pulmonologist, or both. If indeed a patient is diagnosed with refractory asthma, he or she should be followed closely and collaboratively by his or her primary care physician and an asthma specialist.

References

1. Peters S, Ferguson G, Deniz Y, Reisner C. Uncontrolled asthma: a review of the prevalence, disease burden and options for treatment. *Respiratory Medicine*. 2006;100:1139-1151.
2. Proceedings of the ATS Workshop on Refractory Asthma. Current understanding, recommendations, and unanswered questions. *Am J Respir Crit Care Med*. 2000;162:2341-2351.
3. National Asthma Education and Prevention Program. Expert panel report 3 (EPR-3): guidelines for the diagnosis and management of asthma—summary report 2007. *J Allergy Clin Immunol*. 2007;120(5 Suppl):S94-S138.
4. Humbert M, Beasley R, Ayres J, et al. Benefits of omalizumab as add-on therapy in patients with severe persistent asthma who are inadequately controlled despite best available therapy (GINA 2002 step 4 treatment): INNOVATE. *Allergy*. 2005;60:309-316.
5. Richeldi L, Ferrara G, Fabbri LM, Lasserson TJ, Gibson PG. Macrolides for chronic asthma. *Cochrane Database Sys Rev*. 2005;4:CD002997.
6. Cox G. Bronchial thermoplasty for severe asthma. *Curr Opin Pulm Med*. 2011;17:34-38.

27

How Do I Deal With Asthma Exacerbations in My Office?

Amy Renwick, MD

Remember that any child, regardless of his or her history, may have a life-threatening asthma exacerbation. Asthma can be a variable and unpredictable condition, and even mild patients are at risk. Be sure that your office check-in staff can recognize the basic signs of respiratory distress, so children who present with a severe asthma attack or worsen while in the waiting room can be seen and treated promptly (Table 27-1). Similarly, the medical staff should be available, and the check-in staff should be able to interrupt another visit for this potential emergency without any reproach. These are important triage functions that will serve to keep your patients with respiratory problems safe.

The level of acuity appropriate for office treatment varies widely among individual practices. Know your own limits and the availability and limitations of local resources. If you have a packed schedule and few exam rooms, for instance, you will probably have to decide about disposition of a sick patient early in the visit. If you are miles from the nearest emergency room, you may need to provide nearly emergency room-level care in your office regularly. If you or your office staff members are uncomfortable with acutely ill patients, this will also impact your management. No matter how close you are to the nearest emergency room, your office will need basic equipment to treat life-threatening emergencies regardless of the cause. Having what is needed to treat severe acute asthma should be part of this equipment (Table 27-2). This equipment should be readily available, and the maintenance of an emergency cart should be part of the ongoing office routine.

As part of the initial rapid patient assessment, important points in the history include the circumstances of symptom onset, possible triggers, and other exposures. Review with the patient and family any medication(s) used at home, including the frequency of doses and the time(s) of the most recent dose. Finally, quickly ask about the frequency and severity of past asthma exacerbations. Severe croup, anaphylaxis, and possible foreign-body aspiration are other causes of acute respiratory distress that should be

Table 27-1

Reception Desk Red Flags for a Potential Respiratory Emergency

- Labored breathing
- Poor color
  - Pallor
  - Cyanosis
- Audible noisy breathing
- Altered mental status
- Agitation in the parent or child

Table 27-2

Considerations for a Pediatric Office Asthma Emergency Kit

Medications	Oxygen	Medication Delivery Devices

• Albuterol
  ○ Nebulization solution
  ○ Metered-dose inhalers
• Corticosteroids
  ○ Oral
  ○ Inhaled
• Epinephrine
  ○ For severe asthma with poor air entry
  ○ Anaphylaxis
• Ipratropium bromide
  ○ Can be considered for initial therapy in severe asthma
	• Masks and nasal cannulae
	• Ensure that tanks are full
		• Compressors
		• Nebulizers with mouthpieces and masks
		• Valved-holding chambers with mouthpiece and mask

considered in the immediate differential diagnosis and differentiated from an asthma exacerbation as part of this initial assessment.

To gauge the severity of an attack, measure heart rate, respiratory rate, and oxygen saturation, if possible; auscultate for airflow and wheezing; and assess the degree of respiratory effort, including accessory muscle use, shortness of breath, and tolerance of exertion. An asthma scoring system can be implemented if it is practical. Peak flow measurements are useful if the child is already accustomed to the technique.

Inhaled short-acting beta-2-agonists, such as albuterol, are the mainstay of treatment. Give the beta-agonist via a nebulizer or a metered-dose inhaler with spacer/valved-holding chamber, using a mask for children younger than 4 years old and others who cannot use a mouthpiece. (Oral albuterol is not recommended.) Oxygen is also a bronchodilator, and inhaled medications can be delivered with oxygen, if available, directly from a tank or from wall oxygen.

Mild exacerbations may only require a single dose of beta-agonist during the visit. For moderate or severe attacks, beta-agonist can be given in the office every 20 minutes for 3 doses, then every 1 to 4 hours. This protocol is similar to that which would be implemented in an emergency department. Similarly, ipratropium bromide can be administered as part of this initial therapy, if it is available. Monitor heart rate when giving frequent treatments, keeping in mind that tachycardia at presentation often reflects respiratory effort and improves as the medication relieves distress. Provide supplemental oxygen as needed to maintain oxygen saturation of at least 90% to 92%. Occasionally, the oxygen saturation will fall after administration of beta-agonist bronchodilators. This is thought to be due to the positive inotropic effects of these medications, which increases cardiac output and can thereby increase ventilation-perfusion mismatch in the lung.

Systemic steroids are appropriate for children who have already been receiving frequent beta-agonist at home without improvement, who are requiring beta-agonist more often than every 4 hours, or who present with moderate to severe symptoms. Oral prednisone or prednisolone is generally given, at an initial dose of 2 mg/kg (maximum 60 mg), then 1 to 2 mg/kg/day for 3 to 10 days. When a child needs an oral steroid in the office, give the dose as soon as possible, because it will be up to 4 hours before an effect is seen. It is helpful to provide a food or beverage with a pleasant taste after the dose to reduce vomiting, if the degree of respiratory distress is not too severe. Stock a soft solid, such as pudding, to serve as a vehicle for crushed tablets of prednisone when needed for patients who cannot swallow pills or tolerate prednisolone. Dexamethasone, at doses of 0.4 mg/kg to 0.6 mg/kg (maximum 16 to 18 mg), has been used as an alternative and is somewhat more palatable, but studies of its use are limited. It is prudent to screen for recent exposure to varicella before giving a steroid.

Children who present in significant respiratory distress and who do not respond promptly to beta-agonist therapy should be referred to an emergency department or inpatient setting. Reduced initial oxygen saturation—below 94%—also makes it more likely that a child will have ongoing symptoms requiring medical care or hospitalization. More significant reductions in oxygen saturation levels, especially if it is 91% or lower, make this even more likely.

A child with symptoms that are mild, are relieved quickly by beta-agonist, and are expected to be controlled by beta-agonist no more often than every 3 to 4 hours at home (with or without the addition of systemic steroid) can be sent home.

To help determine disposition for other children, check pulse oximetry, and assess symptoms again after 1 hour of treatment. Oxygen saturation 94% or lower is predictive of a need for hospitalization, as is persistence of moderate to severe symptoms. Decisions about whether a child with ongoing symptoms should be transferred by ambulance or by car for further medical treatment should be made individually and conservatively. When in doubt, err on the side of caution.

For children who are well enough to go home, provide clear instructions on medication use and the warning signs that should prompt a return to medical attention. Address any factors that contributed to the severity, such as delay in treatment due to misplaced equipment or expired medication at home, and review correct techniques for using delivery devices. Consider adding inhaled corticosteroids to the regimen for better long-term control. Update the asthma action plan if necessary, and discuss measures to prevent further exacerbations.

References

1. American Academy of Pediatrics Committee on Emergency Medicine. Preparation for emergencies in the offices of pediatric and pediatric primary care providers. *Pediatrics.* 2007;120:200-212.
2. Santillanes G, Gausche-Hill M, Sosa B. Preparedness of selected pediatric offices to respond to critical emergencies in children. *Pediatr Emerg Care.* 2006;22:694-698.
3. Toback SL. Medical emergency preparedness in office practice. *Am Fam Physician.* 2007;75:1679-1684.

HOW CAN I DEAL WITH ASTHMA SYMPTOMS OVER THE TELEPHONE SAFELY AND EFFICIENTLY?

Concettina (Tina) Tolomeo, DNP, APRN, FNP-BC, AE-C

The shortage of primary-care providers[1] coupled with changing consumer and health plan expectations[2] have contributed to the need for telephone care. In parallel, parts of the country are experiencing shortages of subspecialists, which, coupled with the current asthma epidemic, has had a similar effect in terms of access and the need for telephone care. Telephone services in a primary-care practice setting include triage and advice, disease/case management, medication refills/changes, acute illness management, test result interpretation, counseling, and education.[2] Telephone care is one method used for increasing access to care. Ready access to care and advice are important for all parents who have a child with asthma. In addition to practicing self-management by following the agreed-upon written asthma action plan, parents need to feel confident that they can call someone when the plan is not working or when they feel uncomfortable. Safe, quality care and advice for parents of children with asthma should be the goal of telephone triage. Furthermore, providing this type of service efficiently is a necessity in a busy office practice.

Safety and efficiency in the area of telephone management are dependent upon a number of factors. For safety, you must ensure that a qualified person is triaging the phone calls and that a responsive physician is identified and available in the event the telephone point person has any questions. A review of telephone triage and advice studies focusing on nurses' experiences with telephone care revealed that telenurses felt a strong clinical knowledge base was necessary when making assessments via the telephone and that interactions with colleagues increased their assessment skills.[1] Thus, someone with a health-care background is an ideal candidate for such a telephone triage role. In fact, in the primary-care setting, it is the office nurse who is typically given the responsibility of triaging patient phone calls. This choice is fitting if the nurse has training and experience with asthma care and management. Having a health care background alone does not equate to being knowledgeable about asthma care and management. In a study conducted to characterize what nurses working in a primary-care setting know about asthma care, researchers found that many (about 90%) office nurses were unable to identify inflammation of the airways as the underlying problem, and few (about 35%) were aware of the National Asthma Education and Prevention Program (NAEPP) *Guidelines for the Diagnosis and Management of Asthma.*[3]

Another suitable choice for the telephone triage role is a nationally certified asthma educator. Nationally certified asthma educators come from a variety of health-care backgrounds, including, but not limited to, nurses, nurse practitioners, and respiratory therapists. The key is finding a certified asthma educator who best meets the needs of your office practice. For example, if you also need someone to perform office spirometry, a respiratory therapist might be the perfect candidate to fill both roles. This notion may be more fitting for a subspecialty practice, but a nurse with certification as an asthma educator can assume multiple roles in a primary-care setting as well.

In addition to the requisite education and experience level, the person answering the calls must have the ability to gather a thorough history and understanding of the situation at hand. This critical information will allow the determination of the appropriate diagnosis and course of action. Having an algorithm for asthma-related phone calls helps to ensure that all of the essential points are covered in a safe and efficient manner. Additionally, research demonstrates that telenurses value having protocols to help them make decisions. Asthma-related phone call algorithms can also be used to help meet NAEPP guidelines.[4]

When developing an algorithm for your practice, you must keep in mind that the nature of the call will dictate the questions asked. Thus, you may need more than one asthma phone call algorithm, or the algorithm may need to have more than one focal pathway. Moreover, you should take into consideration that the primary motive for an asthma phone call may be disguised by a variety of requests. Therefore, your algorithm needs to account for such instances. For example, a parent may call the office requesting a refill of albuterol, but further questioning and a review of the child's medical record reveals frequent need for the short-acting beta-agonist. Consequently, a call that comes in as a refill request becomes one where asthma symptoms are discussed and a follow-up appointment is scheduled. This example highlights the fact that even short interactions over the telephone should be viewed as teachable moments. Figure 28-1 provides an example of an asthma medication refill request algorithm developed for a pediatric primary-care office.[4]

A refill request is just one of the common reasons parents of children with asthma will call your office. Requesting an appointment and reporting symptoms are two other common reasons. Again, all calls require a different line of questioning to determine the real root of the call.

Finally, in regard to safety, you must remember the importance and necessity of the medical record and timely, accurate documentation. It is imperative that the person triaging phone calls has access to medical records so that the child's health and telephone history can be reviewed. Furthermore, the person triaging the call must document all necessary components of the call—this includes the reason for the call, the education provided, the recommendation provided, the rationale for the recommendation, and the parent's understanding of the education and recommendation provided. A plan for follow-up should be documented as well.

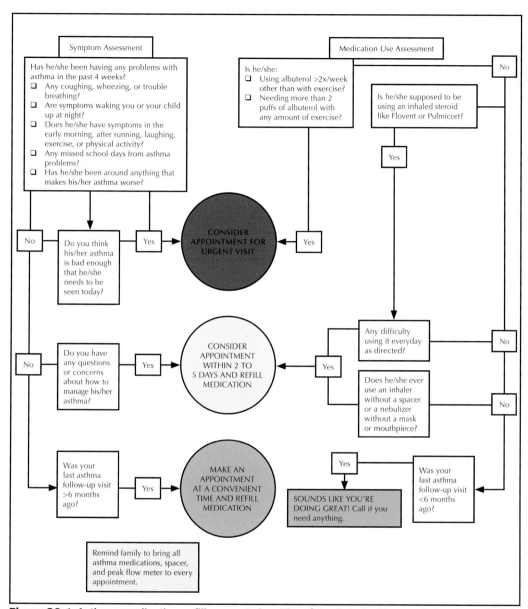

Figure 28-1. Asthma medication refill request algorithm. (Reprinted with permission from Corjulo MT. Telephone triage for asthma medication refills. *Pediatric Nursing.* 2005;31:116-120,124. With permission of Jannetti Publications, Inc.)

How calls can be answered efficiently depends on the size of the practice and the volume of calls. In addition to instituting an asthma algorithm, some practices are so large that they need to employ a person whose sole job is triaging patient phone calls. Such a position allows the person triaging the calls the ability to take the calls as they arrive and address them in real time. If the person triaging the calls is doing so as a part of a larger role (ie, providing education in the office setting), he or she will need some assistance in screening phone calls. Usually, refill and routine appointment requests are not urgent and can be saved for the end of the day. However, it is important to keep in mind that sometimes these types of calls are masking a more urgent problem. Therefore, at the very least, anyone who is calling to schedule an appointment or request a refill should be asked the following question by the office administrative staff: Is your child having symptoms? If the answer is no, the call is best saved to the end of the day when there is protected time for the calls to be answered without interruptions. If the child is having symptoms, the person responsible for triaging calls should take the call immediately and determine if respiratory distress is present. If respiratory distress is present, the parent should be instructed to seek medical attention. If it is not present, the person triaging the call should ask what symptoms are present, how long they have been present, what measures have been taken to relieve the symptoms, and what the response was to the measures taken. The answers to these questions will determine the need for a change in medication therapy and/or the need for an appointment.

Summary

Telephone triage is a necessity in both primary-care and subspecialty office practices. The primary goals are quality and safety. If the person triaging the phone call has any doubt, he or she should have the child evaluated in the office or emergency department. Efficiency is important, but should come second to safety.

References

1. Purc-Stephenson RJ, Thrasher C. Nurses' experiences with telephone triage and advice: a meta-ethnography. *Journal of Advanced Nursing.* 2010;66:482-494.
2. American Academy of Pediatrics Section on Telephone Care and Committee on Child Health Financing. Payment for telephone care. *Pediatrics.* 2006;118:1768-1773.
3. Janson S, Weiss K. What nurses in primary care practices know about asthma care: results from a national survey. *Journal of Asthma.* 2002;39:667-671.
4. Corjulo MT. Telephone triage for asthma medication refills. *Pediatric Nursing.* 2005;31:116-120,124.

WHAT IS INTERMITTENT ASTHMA?

Aaron S. Chidekel, MD

Intermittent asthma is the mildest form of asthma, but it is not a type of asthma that is completely risk-free.[1] In fact, in the most recent asthma guidelines, the "mild" qualifier that previously was associated with intermittent asthma has been removed to emphasize this very point. However, in intermittent asthma, impairment will be low or absent, and airway symptoms will be infrequent (Table 29-1). In fact, because asthma is defined as a disease of chronic airway inflammation, in some ways, the notion of intermittent asthma is something of a paradox. After all, how can a patient have intermittent, chronic airway inflammation? Clearly, intermittent asthma does exist, and depending upon the patient population in your practice, you may see it frequently or infrequently. Still, many patients will have this form of asthma because milder forms of asthma are most common, and these mild patients will require ongoing clinical follow-up, appropriate medical management, and, as with more severely asthmatic patients, a clear action plan to follow.

To address the paradox of airway inflammation in intermittent asthma, it is helpful to consider patients with intermittent asthma as individuals whose airway inflammation has not reached a certain critical threshold to result in the more significant burden of symptoms or lung function abnormalities that are seen in persistent asthma. The level of airway inflammation they experience may be truly intermittent, but it is more likely that it is mild enough that the patient has minimal and intermittent symptoms of asthmatic airway inflammation: cough, wheeze, and mucous production. Similarly, the airways of these patients are not sufficiently inflamed to result in detectable abnormalities on lung function testing, and the risk of airway remodeling is minimal. As normal lung function does not eliminate the presence of truly persistent asthma, spirometry should be followed over time to ensure that the patient's level of lung function remains normal.

Individuals with intermittent asthma will have minimal symptoms. This is often defined in asthma guidelines in the United States as having to use a rescue inhaler less

---

Table 29-1

Cardinal Features of Intermittent Asthma

- Impairment domain
  - Daytime symptoms less than twice weekly
  - Night-time awakenings less than twice monthly
  - Normal activity levels
  - Short-acting beta-agonist use less than twice weekly for rescue
  - Normal lung function
- Risk domain
  - Few or no exacerbations requiring oral corticosteroids

---

than twice weekly during waking hours and less than twice per month to treat nocturnal symptoms/awakenings. Any level of symptoms that is greater than this will no longer fit with the definition of intermittent asthma and will need to be treated with daily controller medication. Similar to this low level of impairment, patients with intermittent asthma will have low levels of risk associated with their condition. They will have infrequent periods of increased symptoms, and these "flares" will not result in the need for oral corticosteroid therapy or emergency asthma care more than once per year. Individuals with intermittent asthma may have exercise-induced bronchospasm and use a short-acting bronchodilator, such as albuterol, prior to exercise to prevent asthma symptoms. Even when used frequently in this fashion, a patient will still meet the criteria for intermittent asthma as long as he or she is not using the short-acting bronchodilator for rescue. It is straightforward and important to quantify these parameters in an asthma follow-up visit and to track them over time in any individual patient to ensure good control of intermittent asthma.

The evaluation of a patient with intermittent asthma will mirror that of a patient with more significant asthma. The likelihood of asthma-related co-morbidities remains, and it is prudent to screen for these as indicated. Atopy and allergic rhinitis often accompany intermittent asthma and should be treated with medications and/or environmental control. Ongoing follow-up and clinical monitoring are also recommended to ensure that the patient's asthma is remaining intermittent and well-controlled. Use of symptom scores, asthma assessment tools, and objective measures of lung function (Figures 29-1 and 29-2) are just as much a part of the management of intermittent asthma as for persistent asthma.

The treatment of intermittent asthma is straightforward. A patient should be instructed in the use of a short-acting beta-agonist for airway symptoms, and an asthma action plan is constructed that reflects this.[2] If a patient is not using a short-acting beta-agonist for exercise, his or her need for refills should be minimal, and he or she should be using no more than 1 or 2 inhalers per year. More frequent requests for medication refills should raise the possibility of more persistent asthma with under-reporting of symptoms, and the patient should be re-assessed. Some patients may also have a prescription for an inhaled corticosteroid to use during brief periods of increased symptoms, but this recommendation is somewhat controversial.[3,4] If a patient requires more than this level of medical management, then he or she is stepped up to a persistent level of asthma, and his or her care plan is adjusted to reflect this change.

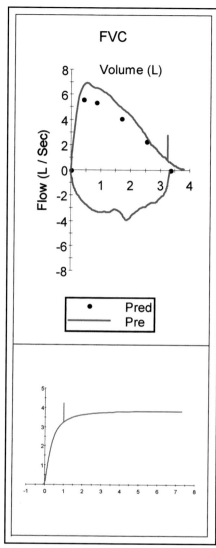

Figure 29-1. Representative flow-volume loop (spirometry) from a patient with intermittent asthma showing a normal flow-volume loop with normal predicted values for age.

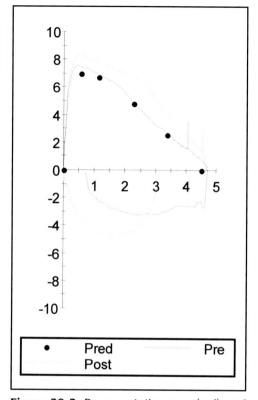

Figure 29-2. Representative pre- (red) and post- (blue) bronchodilator spirometry from a patient with intermittent asthma demonstrating normal to supra-normal flows and volumes. Bronchial hyper-reactivity is indicated pictorially by the increased size of the flow-volume loop in the post-bronchodilator effort.

The prognosis of intermittent asthma is excellent. While most individuals with intermittent asthma tend to stay intermittent, this must not give the patient or physician a false sense of security. Patients still need asthma education and an action plan for periods of wellness as well as in the event of a severe flare. Finally, just like patients with more significant asthma burden, individuals with intermittent asthma need and deserve ongoing follow-up to ensure their continued safety, asthma control, and good health.

References

1. Shahid N, Fitzgerald JM. Current recommendations for the treatment of mild asthma. *J Asthma Allergy.* 2010;3:169-176.
2. Boushey HA, Sorkness CA, King TS, et al. Daily versus as-needed corticosteroids for mild persistent asthma. *N Engl J Med.* 2005;352:1519-1528.
3. National Asthma Education and Prevention Program. *Expert panel report 3 (EPR-3): guidelines for the diagnosis and management of asthma.* Bethesda, MD: National Heart, Lung, and Blood Institute, 2007. NIH publication no. 08-4051.
4. Turpeinen M, Nikander K, Pelkonen AS, et al. Daily versus as-needed inhaled corticosteroid for mild persistent asthma (The Helsinki early intervention childhood asthma study). *Arch Dis Child.* 2008;93:654-659.

WHAT IS PERSISTENT ASTHMA?

Aaron S. Chidekel, MD

Persistent asthma is a broad diagnosis that encompasses children with mild and occasional asthma symptoms to those with debilitating symptoms, severe exacerbations, and asthma that is difficult to control. Examples depicting the different levels of persistent asthma are given in this chapter and summarized in Table 30-1 and Table 30-2. To reflect this diversity of disease severity, asthma guidelines characterize persistent asthma along a continuum or in a stepwise fashion. In the United States asthma guidelines, intermittent asthma is defined as "Step 1" whereas the broad spectrum of persistent asthma is composed of Steps 2 to 6. The guidelines are also stratified by the age of the child with separate management paradigms for children aged 0 to 4 years, 5 to 11 years, and 12 years and older. Whatever the age of the child and wherever the patient falls on this "stepladder of persistent asthma," however, the important characteristic that is shared by all children with persistent asthma is that the need for a daily controller medication is assumed and recommended in the guidelines.

Daily controller therapy is required because children with persistent asthma have chronic airway inflammation that is severe enough to become clinically apparent in a more regular and meaningful fashion. This airway inflammation will be sufficient enough to result in more frequent symptoms and a higher risk of asthma exacerbations. The level of impairment and risk in persistent asthma will be greater than in patients with intermittent asthma (Step 1) and will vary depending upon whether the child has mild (Step 2 to 3), moderate (Step 3 to 4), or severe persistent asthma (Step 5 to 6). Similarly, spirometry or peak flow measurements will begin to detect abnormalities that will vary with the severity, or "step level," of the patient. While the goal is to maintain or to re-establish normal lung function at any level of asthma severity, this becomes more challenging at each level of asthma severity. Lung function measurements are a critical tool for the diagnosis, stratification, and ongoing monitoring of asthma patients, and spirometry is

Table 30-1

Cardinal Features of Persistent Asthma

- Impairment domain
  - Daytime symptoms more than twice weekly
  - Night-time awakenings more than twice monthly
  - Activity levels impacted by asthma with increasing frequency
  - Short-acting beta-agonist use more than twice weekly for rescue
  - Abnormal lung function may be evident
- Risk domain
  - Occurrence of exacerbations requiring oral corticosteroids
  - Abnormal lung function

Table 30-2

Selected Features of Persistent Asthma in Young Children

	Mild	*Moderate*	*Severe*
Children 0 to 4 Years			
Daytime symptoms	Less than 2/week	Everyday	Throughout the day
Nighttime symptoms	Less than 2/month	~Weekly	More than weekly
Activity intolerance	Mild	Moderate	Severe
Need for rescue medication	2 to 7 days/week	Daily	Throughout the day
Children 5 to 11 Years			
Daytime symptoms	Less than 2/week	Everyday	Throughout the day
Nighttime symptoms	Weekly	2 to 7 days/week	May be nightly
Activity intolerance	Mild	Moderate	Severe
Need for rescue medication	2 to 7 days/week	Daily	Throughout the day
FEV1 or peak flow	>80%	60% to 80%	<60%

Adapted from National Asthma Education and Prevention Program. *Expert panel report 3: guidelines for the diagnosis and management of asthma.* Bethesda, MD: National Heart, Lung, and Blood Institute, 2007. NIH publication no. 08-4051.

the test of choice. Examples of spirometry studies from patients with different step levels of persistent asthma are depicted in Figures 30-1 through 30-4. To add to this complexity, because asthma is often a variable and unpredictable disease, children with persistent asthma will move between these steps depending upon their level of asthma control, risk, and current level of symptom severity (impairment). This variability highlights the need for ongoing clinical monitoring and follow-up and the establishment of clear asthma action plans for patients to follow.

At the initial clinical assessment, the child will be "assigned" to a level of asthma severity based upon his or her asthma history and any lung function data (spirometry or peak flow) that are available prior to the initiation of asthma therapy. In general, it is assumed that a child with persistent asthma at the very least will experience asthma symptoms more than twice weekly during waking hours and more than twice per month during the night-time/sleeping hours. Similarly, a patient with intermittent asthma who has had more than one or two exacerbations during the past year should be "stepped up" to a higher (persistent) level of asthma therapy. Finally, patients with abnormal lung function at baseline will also meet the criteria for persistent asthma and should be treated accordingly with a controller medication. Patients who have more frequent or severe symptoms and who have lower levels of baseline lung function will be assigned a higher level of severity and will need to be treated more intensively. At all levels of severity and whatever the age of the child, the preferred initial therapy for persistent asthma is a low dose of an inhaled corticosteroid. Patients may be stepped up to higher levels of therapy with different doses and combinations of controller medications, but the foundation of therapy of persistent asthma is an inhaled corticosteroid for daily control and a short-acting bronchodilator for rescue/symptom relief. Asthma guidelines also suggest the consideration of consultation with an asthma specialist for patients with more significant levels of persistent asthma (see Question 49). Once the patient is assessed and "assigned to a step level of severity," the initial asthma action plan for the patient is then constructed based upon his or her level of symptoms, peak expiratory flow rate (if incorporated), and the initial therapies prescribed.

Individuals with persistent asthma require regular asthma follow-up in order to monitor their level of asthma control and risk. In fact, once the child has been diagnosed with persistent asthma of a certain level of severity, the focus of disease management becomes attaining sufficient "asthma control" and minimizing "asthma risk." Defining asthma control is fairly straightforward. Children should have minimal troublesome symptoms; normal or near-normal levels of lung function, and normal activity levels; and be free of exacerbations requiring oral steroids, emergency care, or hospitalization. "Sleep, school, play" is a simple way to categorize asthma control in children: they should be sleeping well, be attending school regularly, and be free to play normally and as intensely as their nonasthmatic peers.

Another way to think about the goals of asthma control is that the successful medical plan of a patient with persistent asthma should result in a burden of asthma symptoms that is equivalent to intermittent asthma, albeit through the use of controller medications. Defining asthma risk is similarly straightforward. Patients should be free of episodes of status asthmaticus and should have milder exacerbations, and medications should be titrated to avoid side effects from over-medication or inadequate asthma control due to under-medication. In fact, the asthma guidelines suggest that therapy be

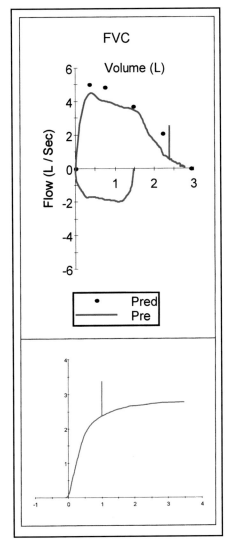

Figure 30-1. This is a representative pre-bronchodilator flow-volume loop (spirometry) from a patient with "Step 2 to 3 asthma" showing a normally configured flow-volume loop with predicted values for age that are at the lower limit of normal.

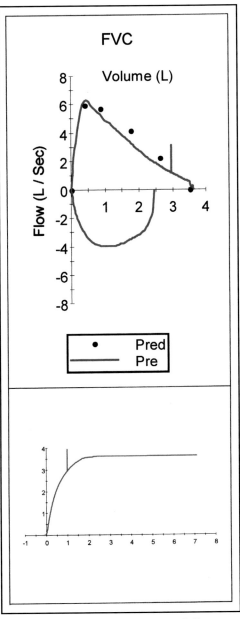

Figure 30-2. This is a representative pre-bronchodilator flow-volume loop (spirometry) from a patient with "Step 3 to 4 asthma" showing a minimally scooped flow-volume loop with normal predicted values for age.

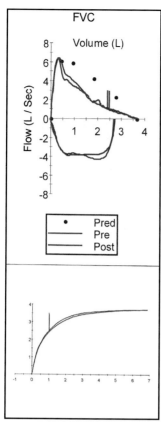

Figure 30-3. This is a representative pre- and post-bronchodilator flow-volume loop (spirometry) from a patient with "Step 4 to 5 asthma" showing significant airway obstruction without a significant response to bronchodilator. This lack of bronchodilator suggests fixed airway obstruction and airway remodeling. Airway remodeling is thought to represent the effects of longstanding airway inflammation on the lung and may be due to airway smooth muscle hypertrophy, basement membrane thickening due to collagen deposition, or other factors.

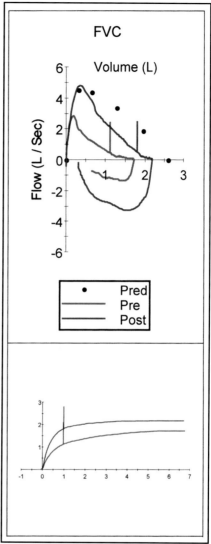

Figure 30-4. This is a representative pre- and post-bronchodilator flow-volume loop (spirometry) from a patient with "Step 5 to 6 asthma" showing severe airway obstruction with marked reversibility. This level of bronchial hyper-reactivity despite ongoing aggressive medical therapy places this patient at high risk for a severe asthma episode and is a difficult challenge.

re-evaluated regularly so the medications can be titrated up if control remains poor or risk remains high or titrated down if asthma control has been achieved and maintained for several months. The management of persistent pediatric asthma is a continuous process of evaluation and follow-up, with ongoing medication adjustments (up or down) depending upon the clinical status of the child.

The medical management of persistent asthma is well-characterized and presented in the most recent asthma guidelines. As already mentioned, the preferred therapy for "Step 2" persistent asthma is a low dose of an inhaled corticosteroid. Alternative treatment options include the leukotriene receptor antagonist montelukast, the nonsteroidal anti-inflammatory agents cromolyn or nedocromil, and theophylline. From a practical stand-point, cromolyn and nedocromil are no longer readily available, and in my own practice, I have not used theophylline in more than 15 years. The preferred treatment of Step 3 persistent asthma in young children (aged 0 to 4 years) is a medium dose of an inhaled corticosteroid. In older children, combinations of a low-dose inhaled corticosteroid and either a long-acting bronchodilator or montelukast (or theophylline) is recommended above an intermediate dose of an inhaled corticosteroid. It is important to be familiar with individual inhaled corticosteroid preparations and their dosages and to be familiar with the "black-box" warning that is associated with medications containing long-acting bronchodilators so that the options can be fully discussed with parents and patients when devising a treatment plan. Allergen immunotherapy is noted as an adjunctive therapy in appropriate patients for persistent asthma in Steps 2 to 4. The management of the "upper steps" (Steps 4 to 6) is more complex with higher doses and different combinations of the available asthma controller medications. As noted, the input of an asthma specialist should be considered for children requiring these higher levels of therapy. Omalizumab enters the step ladder at Step 5 for patients aged 12 years and older, and the other anti-leukotriene agent Zileuton, which inhibits leukotriene synthesis, enters the step ladder at Step 3. Irrespective of where the patient falls in this paradigm, patient education, environmental control, and the diagnosis and management of comorbidities is critical, and the guidelines recommend a "step-up or step-down approach" depending upon the patient's level of control and risk at 3-month intervals.

The prognosis of persistent asthma varies with the individual disease state of the patient. While infants and young children with persistent asthma may still go into remission, the longer that asthma symptoms persist and the more frequent and severe the symptoms, the less likely it is that this will occur. Similarly, those children who develop persistent asthma during childhood are also less likely to experience a remission of their symptoms. Some patients with severe levels of persistent asthma can be quite difficult to manage and control, whereas others, the majority in fact, will respond well to simple controller therapy. Regardless of the level of severity and symptoms experienced by the patient, the goals of therapy are the same: to establish and maintain asthma control and minimize the risk of both the asthma and its therapy so that the child can live a normal and healthy life. Asthma education, the formulation of an individualized action plan, and the monitoring and management of comorbidities are the other critical factors for successful and guideline-centered management.

Suggested Readings

Cornell A, Shaker M, Woodmansee DP. Update on the pathogenesis and management of childhood asthma. *Curr Opin Pediatr.* 2008;20:597-604.

Fanta CH, Carter EL, Stieb ES, Haver KE. *The Asthma Educator's Handbook.* New York, NY: McGraw Hill Medical; 2007.

Lougheed MD, Lemiere C, Dell SD, et al. Canadian Thoracic Society Asthma Management Continuum—2010 Consensus Summary for children six years of age and over, and adults. *Can Respir J.* 2010;17:15-24.

National Asthma Education and Prevention Program. *Expert panel report 3 (EPR-3): guidelines for the diagnosis and management of asthma.* Bethesda, MD: National Heart, Lung, and Blood Institute, 2007. NIH publication no. 08-4051.

Potter PC. Current guidelines for the management of asthma in young children. *Allergy Asthma Immunol Res.* 2010;2:1-13.

HOW IS EXERCISE-INDUCED ASTHMA DIAGNOSED AND TREATED?

Brad Bley, DO, CSCS and Aaron S. Chidekel, MD

As noted previously, asthma is characterized by reversible airway obstruction, hyper-responsiveness, and inflammation with the typical symptoms of shortness of breath, cough, wheezing, and chest tightness. As the term implies, exercise-induced broncho-spasm (EIB) occurs during exercise and may exist in individuals with and without a known history of asthma. Even when asthma is well-controlled on inhaled corticoste-roids, a majority of patients with persistent asthma may still have exercise-induced asth-ma (EIA). The exact prevalence of EIB in the general population is unknown, but various studies have reported a prevalence ranging from 6% to 29%.[1-4] This wide range is likely due to a variety of testing techniques, patient populations, and disagreement on the per-centage decrease in forced expiratory volume in one second (FEV1) that should be used to make a diagnosis of EIA. For example, normal children can have a postexercise decrease in peak expiratory flow rate (PEFR) as high as 15%,[5,6] so a decrease in FEV1 greater than 15% is typically used to diagnose EIA, but some studies have used a decrease in FEV1 greater than 10%. All of these factors can complicate the diagnosis of EIB and/or EIA.

Differentiating between EIB, EIA, and other causes of dyspnea in an athlete or even the non-athlete can be difficult. The differential diagnosis for exercise-induced dyspnea (EID) is broad and includes exercise-induced laryngeal dysfunction (vocal cord dysfunction [VCD] or exercise-induced laryngomalacia), exercise-induced gastroesophageal reflux, exercise-induced postnasal drip, exercise-induced hyperventilation, deconditioning, physiologic exercise limitation, costochondritis, chest pain, restrictive physiology, cardiac arrhythmias, and pulmonary or cardiac shunts (Table 31-1).

The sensation of dyspnea is subjective and different for everyone. Dyspnea is the per-ception of difficulty or painful breathing and is a common experience with exercise but is also a symptom of a multitude of medical disorders. Syncope needs to be differenti-ated from dyspnea immediately in the history, and exercise-induced syncope is a major

Table 31-1

The Differential Diagnosis of Exercise-Induced Dyspnea in Children

- Exercise-induced laryngeal dysfunction
  - Vocal cord dysfunction
  - Exercise-induced laryngomalacia
- Post-nasal drip
- Gastroesophageal reflux
- Hyperventilation
- Deconditioning
- Physiologic exercise limitation
- Costochondritis
- Restrictive chest wall disorders
  - Pectus excavatum
- Cardiac disease (often presents with syncope)
  - Idiopathic hypertrophic cardiomyopathy
  - Prolonged QTc syndrome
  - Anomalous coronary artery
  - Other congenital heart disease

red flag. Children with exercise-induced syncope should have their activities curtailed and need to be promptly evaluated for an underlying cardiac disease, such as idiopathic hypertrophic cardiomyopathy or prolonged QTc syndrome. Psychological factors may also play an important role in the sensation of dyspnea.[7] In addition, it is often difficult for patients to identify whether their fatigue or dyspnea is due to "being out of shape," a correctable organic cause such as those already mentioned, or the natural limit of their ability. In the office, distinguishing a deconditioned patient or a physically fit athlete who has reached his or her physiologic exercise limitation, both common and natural causes of exercise intolerance, from other organic etiologies can be just as difficult. Even among competitive and elite athletes, recognizing those with EIA can be difficult. Before the 1984 Olympic Games, the US Olympic committee evaluated its athletes and found that 67 of 597 members tested positive for EIA, while only 26 had been previously identified as having EIA.[8]

To complicate matters even more, it is not uncommon for there to be multiple causes of EID occurring at the same time. Several recent studies have attempted to evaluate the accuracy of the clinical diagnosis of EIA. In one such study, Abu-Hasan and colleagues looked at children referred to a pediatric allergy and pulmonary clinic and found that only 11 of 117 patients who experienced symptoms during an exercise stress test had EIA (defined as a decrease in FEV1 of greater than or equal to 15%).[4] In a similar fashion, Seear and colleagues evaluated 52 children who were referred for poorly controlled EIA and found that only 2 fulfilled the same diagnostic criteria for EIA.[5] However, both of these studies were performed at major referral centers and likely represent a different patient population than most practicing physicians will encounter in their office. If

---

Table 31-2

Potential Testing to Evaluate Exercise Intolerance

- Spirometry
- Complete pulmonary function testing
- Cardiopulmonary exercise testing
- Cardiopulmonary exercise testing with laryngoscopy
- Bronchoprovocation testing
- Electrocardiogram
- Echocardiogram
- Holter monitoring

---

anything, these studies are important reminders that every patient who presents with EID will not necessarily have a diagnosis of EIA and that the differential diagnosis of EID is much broader. Evaluation and treatment of such patients require, like most illnesses in medicine, a thorough history and physical examination. Additional testing can then be performed based upon the specific needs of the patient. Testing options are presented in Table 31-2.

Of note, the first step in this testing includes spirometry. However, if clinical suspicion of EIB is high, a short trial of a bronchodilator is likely to be much more cost effective than ordering spirometry for every patient who presents with EID to the primary-care office. If symptoms do not improve, however, spirometry should be considered before the addition of other medications. If spirometry reveals evidence of airway obstruction with a decrease in FEV1, decreased mid-expiratory flows, and a reduced FEV1 to forced vital capacity (FVC) ratio, then the diagnosis of persistent asthma is suggested and should be treated as the first step. Similarly, normal spirometry does not completely eliminate the possibility of asthma, and therefore additional testing may be required. If additional testing is required, it is important to remember that physiologic documentation is particularly important because of the subjective nature of the complaint of dyspnea and to "rule in" or "rule out" other less common medical diagnoses that may be associated with adverse outcomes. In addition, patients may have overlapping conditions concurrently. Treatment, while generally straightforward, needs to be related to the results of testing and the response to any treatment to date to avoid unnecessary over- or under-medication.

As many as 30% of young people with asthma limit their activity compared with just 5% of children without asthma.[9] In the era of ever-expanding waistlines, the promotion of physical activity at a young age is becoming more and more important. The primary aim of therapy in patients with isolated EIB is prophylaxis, while the primary aim of therapy in those patients with asthma and concurrent EIA is overall asthma control with elimination of exercise as one of the patient's triggers and then the additional prophylaxis of EIB, if required. Treatment starts with the optimization of therapy for underlying persistent asthma, and the importance of this cannot be emphasized strongly enough. As discussed previously, particular attention should be given to differentiating between patients with isolated EIB and those with asthma and EIA.

Table 31-3

Recommended Interventions for Exercise-Induced Bronchospasm

- Nonmedical interventions
  - ○ Warm-up period prior to exercise
  - ○ Cool-down period after exercise
  - ○ Maintain nose breathing as much as possible
  - ○ Wear a mask on cold days
  - ○ Monitor indoor and outdoor air quality
- Medical interventions
  - ○ Treat underlying persistent asthma
  - ○ Pre-medicate with short-acting beta-agonist 15 to 30 minutes prior to exercise
  - ○ May repeat during exercise with caution

Nonmedical therapies for EIB are critical and effective in reducing its occurrence and severity (Table 31-3). These include attending to environmental factors, such as ambient temperature, air quality, and the exercise environment, remembering that ice rinks, some swimming pools, and dusty gymnasiums may be especially problematic. Prior to exercise, it is important to perform a warm up and to cool down after completing the work out. Nose breathing should be emphasized so as to warm and moisten the inspired air as much as possible, and if exercise in cold air cannot be avoided, a mask can be worn. Coaches, gym teachers, and other supervising adults should be alerted to the asthmatic condition of the child, and the appropriate medications, delivery devices, and action plan should be directly on hand at the site of exercise, not in the locker room or in the car.

Medical therapy for EIB is also straightforward and effective. In the patient with underlying asthma and EIA, it begins with the appropriate controller therapy as required by the patient. For both patients with isolated EIB and EIA, the administration of a short-acting beta-agonist 15 to 30 minutes prior to exercise is the treatment of choice. In the past, pretreatment with the nonsteroidal anti-inflammatory agents cromolyn sodium and nedocromil was also recommended; however, these medications are no longer readily available. Montelukast can also blunt EIB and may be an additional agent to consider, particularly in those children with underlying persistent asthma that is mild in nature. The treatment of other comorbidities, such as allergic rhinitis and gastroesophageal reflux, can also improve exercise performance in children with asthma and/or isolated EIB.

Summary

Optimizing exercise performance in all children begins with the thorough and accurate assessment of exercise-related breathing problems. Very high levels of athletic performance are possible, even in children with significant underlying asthma. Unfortunately, however, rare catastrophes have occurred, and the under-diagnosis and under-treatment of asthma in some of these cases likely played a role. In children with dyspnea without syncope, it is rare to find a truly life-threatening comorbidity that will result in activity limitation. Rather, the goal should be to diagnose and treat any element of asthma and then to address any additional element of EIB that is interfering with the ability of the child to run and play normally.

References

1. Randolph C. Exercise-induced asthma: update on pathophysiology, clinical diagnosis, and treatment. *Curr Probl Pediatr.* 1997;27:53-77.
2. Rupp NT, Brudno DS, Guill MF. The value of screening for risk of exercise-induced asthma in high school athletes. *Ann Allergy.* 1993;70:339-342.
3. Mannix ET, Roberts M, Fagin DP, et al. The prevalence of airways hyperresponsiveness in members of an exercise training facility. *J Asthma.* 2003;40:349-355.
4. Rupp NT, Guill MF, Brudno DS. Unrecognized exercise-induced bronchospasm in adolescent athletes. *Am J Dis Child.* 1992;146:941-944.
5. Mehta H, Busse WW. Prevalence of exercise-induced asthma in the athlete. In: Weiler JM, ed. *Allergic and Respiratory Disease in Sports Medicine.* New York, NY: Marcel Dekker, Incorporated; 1997:81-86.
6. Kattan M, Keens TG, Mellis CM, Levison H. The response to exercise in normal and asthmatic children. *J Pediatr.* 1978;92:718-721.
7. Weinberger, M, Abu-Hasan, M. Perceptions and pathophysiology of dyspnea and exercise intolerance. *Pediatr Clin N Am.* 2009;56:33-48.
8. Voy RO. The US Olympic Committee experience with exercise-induced bronchospasm. *Med Sci Sports Exerc.* 1986;18:328-330.
9. Taylor W, Newacheck P. Impact of childhood asthma on health. *Pediatrics.* 1992;90:657-662.

Suggested Readings

Abu-Hasan M, Tannous B, Weinberger M. Exercise-induced dyspnea in children and adolescents: if not asthma then what? *Ann Allergy Asthma Immunol.* 2005;94:366-371.

Becker JM, Rogers J, Rossini G, Mirchandani H, D'Alonzo GE Jr. Asthma deaths during sports: report of a 7-year experience. *J Allergy Clin Immunol.* 2004;113:264-267.

Cava JR, Danduran MJ, Fedderly RT, Sayger PL. Exercise recommendations and risk factors for sudden cardiac death. *Pediatr Clin North Am.* 2004;51:1401-1420.

Heinle R, Linton A, Chidekel AS. Exercise-induced vocal cord dysfunction presenting as asthma in pediatric patients: toxicity of inappropriate inhaled corticosteroids and the role of exercise laryngoscopy. *Pediatr Asthma Allergy Immunol.* 2003;16:215-224.

Parsons JP, Mastronarde JG. Exercise-induced bronchoconstriction in athletes. *Chest.* 2005;128:3966-3974.

Seear M, Wensley D, West N. How accurate is the diagnosis of exercise induced asthma among Vancouver schoolchildren? *Arch Dis Child.* 2005;90:898-902.

Storms WW. Exercise-induced asthma in athletes: current issues. *J Asthma.* 1995;32:245-257.

Turcotte H, Langdeau JB, Thibault G, Boulet LP. Prevalence of respiratory symptoms in an athlete population. *Respir Med.* 2003;97:955-963.

Weinberger M, Abu-Hasan M. Perceptions and pathophysiology of dyspnea and exercise intolerance. *Pediatr Clin North Am.* 2009;56:33-48.

SECTION VI

ASTHMA EMERGENCY AND INPATIENT CARE

WHAT IS STATUS ASTHMATICUS?
WHO IS AT RISK FOR IT AND
WHAT ARE ITS CAUSES?

Jonathan E. Bennett, MD and Aaron S. Chidekel, MD

Status asthmaticus is defined differently among authors. Probably the most useful definition is that it is a severe asthma exacerbation that does not respond to initial bronchodilator therapy and that may become life threatening. This definition reinforces the role of inflammation in asthma and the notion that the inflammatory response needs to be treated differently from acute bronchospasm. From the standpoint of the most recent asthma guidelines that highlight the notion of asthma control and risk, status asthmaticus also represents an acute episode during which control is at a nadir and risk is at a peak. Status asthmaticus is a common and important occurrence, and asthma remains a very common reason for hospitalization and emergency department visits for children.

Status asthmaticus is typically triggered, as in less severe asthma attacks, by upper respiratory tract infections, environmental allergens and irritants, or exercise. Occasionally, no trigger is identified. Another subgroup of patients have what is termed *brittle asthma*, which is asthma that has deteriorated and become more unstable over a longer period of time, days to weeks. Brittle asthma is also a risk factor for an episode of status asthmaticus occurring. More frequent symptoms, diurnal peak flow variability, and worsened nocturnal asthma are all clues that a patient's asthma control is slipping and that asthma is becoming "brittle." An asthma action plan can help a patient recognize when his or her asthma control is slipping and the risk for status asthmaticus is increasing. This can then be followed up with a visit to the physician for medication adjustment or other medical or environmental change.

Regarding the issue of who is at risk for status asthmaticus, epidemiologic studies link high rates of asthma hospitalization and the highest death rates with poverty, ethnic minorities, and urban living.[1] This increased risk most likely results from a combination of factors, including biologic vulnerability, increased exposure to airway irritants and allergens, and poor asthma management. Respiratory viral infections are also commonly

Table 32-1

Risk Factors for Death From Asthma

- Asthma history
- Previous severe exacerbation (eg, intubation or intensive care unit admission for asthma)
- 2 or more hospitalizations for asthma in the past year
- 3 or more emergency department visits for asthma in the past year
- Hospitalization or emergency department visit for asthma in the past month
- Using more than 2 canisters of short-acting beta-agonist per month
- Difficulty perceiving asthma symptoms or severity of exacerbations
- Other risk factors: lack of a written asthma action plan, sensitivity to *Alternaria*
- Social history
- Low socioeconomic status or inner-city residence
- Illicit drug use
- Major psychosocial problems
- Comorbidities
- Cardiovascular disease
- Other chronic lung disease
- Chronic psychiatric disease

Adapted from National Asthma Education and Prevention Program. *Expert panel report 3 (EPR-3): guidelines for the diagnosis and management of asthma. Section 5: managing exacerbations of asthma.* Bethesda, MD: National Heart, Lung, and Blood Institute, 2007:373-417.

linked to episodes of status asthmaticus in children. Many of these factors are discussed in increased detail in other questions in this book. It would be very useful to identify those children who are at risk for severe status asthmaticus and especially those at risk for death, but this remains a challenge. Table 32-1 from the National Asthma Education and Prevention *Expert Panel Report 3* lists potential risk factors for fatal asthma attacks. Unfortunately, in studies of fatal asthma cases, potentially preventable elements are frequently not found.[2]

Status asthmaticus occurs when the airway inflammation and bronchospasm associated with underlying asthma lead to sufficient airflow limitation and airway irritation to cause symptoms of coughing, wheezing, and shortness of breath. Changes in lung compliance and lung volumes lead to increased work of breathing. Airway obstruction from bronchospasm, mucous plugging, and airway edema leads to air trapping and lung overinflation. Lung overinflation in turn causes the expiratory phase of breathing to become an active process, and prolonged exhalation and respiratory muscle activity during exhalation become apparent. Patients with status asthmaticus therefore demonstrate increased expiratory work of breathing, and this results in positive intrapleural pressures during exhalation as well. This can have effects on cardiac function, which can be detected by the exaggerated respiratory swings in blood pressure, referred to as pulsus paradoxus. Increasing pulsus paradoxus in status asthmaticus correlates with increasing levels of airflow obstruction.

These changes in airway caliber and tone, lung volumes, and airflow can affect both oxygenation and ventilation. Ventilation-perfusion mismatching is the most common mechanism of the mild hypoxemia that often accompanies status asthmaticus. Increased work of breathing and the shortness of breath experienced by patients often result in mild hyperventilation as well, and it is not uncommon to see mildly reduced levels of carbon dioxide, either in the blood or as measured by capnometry. Mild hypoxemia and respiratory alkalosis are the most common blood-gas abnormalities seen in status asthmaticus that is not too severe. This is why it is often stated that a normal carbon dioxide level during an asthma attack may be of concern. Other alarming blood gas values in status asthmaticus include elevated carbon dioxide levels (respiratory acidosis) and severe hypoxemia, but it is lactic acidosis that is particularly associated with a poor prognosis and extremely high risk of respiratory failure.

Determining the severity of an episode of status asthmaticus takes experience, and the degree of the wheezing that is heard does not correlate well with severity of airflow obstruction. Clearly, a silent chest, in which no airflow is auscultated, is alarming as is the presence of agitation and severe dyspnea. Other clues of impending respiratory failure include altered mental status, inability to speak or lie down, cyanosis, and diaphoresis. Patients with status asthmaticus, particularly young children, can progress rapidly, and careful observation and clinical monitoring are critical, particularly during the initial stages of treatment. Medical management of wheezing in the emergency department setting is discussed in Question 33, and indications for asthma admission are discussed in Question 35.

Summary

One of the most important goals of guideline-driven asthma management is the prevention of episodes of status asthmaticus through the implementation of solid asthma action plans and chronic controller therapy. Identifying patients at high risk for status asthmaticus remains a challenge, and therefore early recognition and medical intervention remain critically important. When an episode of status asthmaticus does occur, aggressive medical therapy and careful clinical patient assessment and monitoring are critical.

References

1. Frederico MJ, Liu AH. Overcoming childhood asthma disparities of the inner city poor. *Ped Clin North Am.* 2003;50:655-675.
2. Robertson CF, Rubinfeld AR, Bowes G. Pediatric asthma deaths in Victoria: the mild are at risk. *Pediatric Pulmonology.* 1992;13:95-100.

Suggested Readings

Chipps BE, Murphy KR. Assessment and management of acute asthma in children. *J Pediatr.* 2006;147:288-294.

National Asthma Education and Prevention Program. *Expert panel report 3 (EPR-3): guidelines for the diagnosis and management of asthma. Section 5: managing exacerbations of asthma.* Bethesda, MD: National Heart, Lung, and Blood Institute, 2007:373-417.

Mannix R, Bachur R. Status asthmaticus in children. *Curr Opin Pediatr.* 2007;19:281-287.

Yock Corrales A, Soto-Martinez M, Starr M. Management of severe asthma in children. *Aust Fam Physician.* 2011;40:35-38.

HOW SHOULD A CHILD WHO PRESENTS TO THE EMERGENCY ROOM WITH WHEEZING BE ASSESSED AND TREATED?

Jonathan E. Bennett, MD

The first consideration when evaluating a wheezing child is whether the wheezing is likely to be asthma or, in the case of a child without prior wheezing, bronchospasm. Some focused questions will allow one to quickly assess the likelihood that the wheezing child is experiencing asthma or bronchospasm:

1. Has the child had previous similar episodes? Recurrent episodes of wheezing are very suggestive of asthma.
2. Do other family members have asthma? A family history of asthma is suggestive of asthma.
3. Was this episode preceded by upper respiratory symptoms? Most asthma attacks are triggered by upper respiratory illnesses.
4. Did the symptoms come on very rapidly, or did they follow an episode of choking or gagging? Rapid onset of wheezing or difficulty breathing may suggest an allergic reaction or, especially with a history of choking or gagging, foreign-body aspiration.
5. Is there a history of cardiac disease or failure to thrive? Congestive heart failure and cystic fibrosis may present with wheezing and may also cause failure to thrive.

Once it is felt the symptoms are due to asthma or bronchospasm, the assessment of the wheezing child is almost exclusively clinical. The first step is to determine the degree of respiratory distress present, as this will dictate how rapid any interventions must be. Respiratory failure, or impending respiratory failure, must be addressed immediately and aggressively. Agitation or lethargy, dusky mucous membranes, minimal air movement, marked accessory muscle use, and oxygen saturation below 90% may all be signs of respiratory failure. In patients without respiratory failure, it is useful to classify patients by degree of severity, as this will also help to tailor management. Table 33-1 shows a useful clinical classification for asthma severity.[1] Scoring systems, such as the Pulmonary Index,[2] have been developed to assign a numerical score based on clinical

Table 33-1

Evaluation of Acute Asthma Exacerbation Severity

Sign/Symptom	Mild	Moderate	Severe
Respiratory rate	Normal to 30% increase	30% to 50% increase	>50% increase
Alertness	Normal or agitated	Normal or agitated	Agitated to decreased level of conciousness
Dyspnea	Absent or mild; speech normal	Moderate; speaks in phrases; difficulty feeding	Severe; single words or phrases; refuses feeding
Accessory muscle use	None to mild intercostal retractions	Moderate intercostal with suprasternal ret; use of sternoclei-domastoid muscle; chest hyperinflation	Severe intercostal and tracheosternal retractions; nasal flaring; chest hyperinflation
Color	Normal	Pale	Possibly cyanotic
Wheeze	Often end expiratory only	Throughout expiration	Throughout inhalation and expiration, breath sounds markedly decreased
Oxygen saturation	>95%	91% to 95%	<91%
Peak expiratory flow rate (% predicted or personal best)	>80%	50% to 80%	<50%
$PaCO_2$	<42 mm Hg	<42 mm Hg	>42 mm Hg

Adapted from National Asthma Education and Prevention Program. *Expert panel report 3 (EPR-3): guidelines for the diagnosis and management of asthma. Section 5: managing exacerbations of asthma.* Bethesda, MD: National Heart, Lung, and Blood Institute, 2007:373-417.

parameters, including some of those found in Table 33-1. In the Pulmonary Index, a score of less than 6 represents a mild asthma exacerbation, while a score of more than 10 represents a severe exacerbation. Scoring systems are most frequently used in research studies to assess severity, but also can be used to develop treatment algorithms and monitor response to therapy.

A peak flow meter may be used to objectively assess airflow obstruction. In general, children ages 6 years and older are cooperative enough and can be instructed in how to perform peak expiratory flow rates (PEFR). This measurement is most useful in patients who perform them regularly at home so that measurements taken during an acute attack can be compared to their personal best PEFR when healthy. There are predicted values available based on gender and height that can be used for children who have not done PEFR or cannot remember their personal best.

There is little role of ancillary testing in wheezing patients. Chest radiographs do little to change management in the asthmatic patient. They should be considered in patients with high fever and focal findings (persistent focal wheezing, focal rales, or decreased breath sounds) that may suggest pneumonia and in patients where there is concern for pneumothorax or pneumomediastinum (severe disease or persistent decreased breath sounds). Chest radiographs should also be considered in first-time wheezing patients, especially when an alternative diagnosis (see Question 34) is being strongly considered. Similarly, arterial blood gas sampling has little value in the emergent management of the wheezing child. Oxygenation can be assessed noninvasively with pulse oximetry. $PaCO_2$ is often elevated in severe illness early in the course of therapy, and its measurement at that time is unlikely to affect management. Although it can be used over time to track deterioration, the decision to intubate is made on a clinical basis.

Once the severity of the episode has been determined, treatment can be tailored appropriately. The mainstay of any wheezing episode thought to be due to bronchospasm is inhaled beta-agonist therapy, such as albuterol. In mild cases, this may be given as individual doses, with reassessment after the doses to determine effect. The dose of nebulized albuterol is generally quoted as 0.15 mg/kg per dose. Many institutions, however, dose albuterol according to broader weight ranges, with children less than 20 kg receiving 2.5 mg per dose and children over 20 kg receiving 5 mg per dose. In moderate to severe cases, which require multiple doses, these doses should be given as either 3 back-to-back treatments over 45 to 60 minutes or as a continuous nebulization over 60 minutes (10 mg/hr in patients 5 to 10 kg, 15 mg/hr in patients 10 to 20 kg, and 20 mg/hr in patients over 20 kg). Moderate to severe cases should also receive two to three doses of inhaled ipratropium bromide, an anticholinergic bronchodilator, over this time period as well. The use of ipratropium bromide in moderate to severe asthma exacerbations has been shown to decrease the need for hospitalization.[3] Traditionally, beta-agonist therapy has been given by nebulization. There is, however, strong evidence that delivery by metered-dose inhaler with spacer (MDI-S) in children is just as effective as nebulization. This route may certainly be used for mild cases. For moderate cases, MDI-S may theoretically be used, although given the need to give ipratropium bromide (which can be given concomitantly with nebulized albuterol), nebulization is often more practical. Another advantage of nebulizer delivery is that, for children with oxygen saturations less than 92%, oxygen can be delivered along with nebulized medications. In the most severe cases, when there is concern about delivery of nebulized medication due to inadequate air movement, subcutaneous terbutaline may be given at a dose of 0.01 mg/kg (maximum 0.4 mg).

Along with initial bronchodilator therapy, moderate to severe cases should receive a dose of steroids. Oral steroids have been shown to be as effective as intravenous steroids and reduce the need for hospitalization. Oral prednisone or prednisolone are given at doses of 1 to 2 mg/kg. Dexamethasone phosphate is an alternative, given at a dose of 0.6 mg/kg (maximum 10 to 12 mg). It may be advantageous to use prednisolone, as the IV formulation (10 mg/mL) can be given orally in a smaller volume, and it has a longer half-life (36 to 72 hours) than prednisone or prednisolone, with similar efficacy. In cases of severe respiratory distress or vomiting, intravenous methylprednisolone should be given at a dose of 1 to 2 mg/kg (maximum 125 mg).

The majority of moderate to severe asthma patients will respond to the measures discussed. For those who do not, there is some evidence that intravenous magnesium sulfate 50 to 75 mg/kg (maximum 2 g) can reduce the need for hospitalization.[4] In the severe cases not responding to continuous inhaled beta-agonist, intravenous terbutaline can also be initiated. This is started with a 5 to 10 mcg/kg bolus followed by a 0.3 to 0.5 mcg/kg/min infusion titrating to effect to a maximum of 5 mcg/kg/min. For the most severe patients who are deteriorating despite maximal therapy, noninvasive positive pressure ventilation may be useful to avoid intubation.

Summary

Most acute episodes of wheezing are due to flares of pre-existing asthma often associated with a respiratory viral infection or exposure to another known trigger. Careful history and physical examination can guide the need for additional testing in a patient with previously diagnosed asthma, and this testing can often be deferred. A new-onset episode of wheezing requires more careful consideration while treatment is initiated. Aggressive medical therapy, as outlined previously, and supplemental oxygen if necessary are often all that are needed to address the flare, and the majority of patients can be discharged home with close clinical follow-up.

References

1. Stevenson MD, Ruddy RM. Asthma and allergic emergencies In: Fleisher GR, Ludwig S, Henretig FM, eds. *Textbook of Pediatric Emergency Medicine*. 6th ed. Philadelphia, PA: Lippincott Williams & Wilkins; 2009.
2. Becker AB, Nelson NA, Simons SE. The pulmonary index. Assessment of a clinical score for asthma. *Am J Dis Child*. 1984;138:574-576.
3. Qureshi F, Pestian J, Davis P, Zaritsky A. Effect of nebulized ipratropium on the hospitalization rates in children. *N Engl J Med*. 1998;339:1030-1035.
4. Chuek DK, Chau DC, Lee SL. A meta-analysis on intravenous magnesium sulphate for treating acute asthma. *Arch Dis Child*. 2005;90:74-77.

WHAT ARE SOME RESPIRATORY EMERGENCIES THAT CAN PRESENT LIKE ASTHMA?

Jonathan E. Bennett, MD

The previous question regarding the treatment of the wheezing child was answered with the presumption that the wheezing was due to asthma or bronchospasm. There is nothing wrong with initiating therapy for a wheezing child before a definitive diagnosis is made, especially a child in respiratory distress. However, it is important to remember that not all wheezing is due to asthma. Wheezing occurs due to intrinsic or extrinsic obstruction of the intrathoracic airways, the bronchioles, or less commonly due to obstruction of the trachea or bronchi. Wheezing is often defined as an expiratory breath sound, whereas stridor is considered to be an inspiratory breath sound. Although this distinction is clearcut on paper, at times, the lines are blurred in the clinical realm, and findings can be concurrent and overlapping. Although wheezing is most commonly due to asthma, there are a number of other causes of airway obstruction that may present like asthma. It is critical to remember these differential diagnostic possibilities, particularly in patients with severe presentations or those with inadequate responses to standard asthma therapies.

By far the most common respiratory emergency that presents like asthma in infants and young children is bronchiolitis. This viral illness, which affects children younger than 2 years of age, is most commonly caused by the respiratory syncytial virus, but can be caused by a number of other respiratory viruses. Viruses such as human metapneumovirus, rhinovirus, and para-influenza have all been associated with the clinical syndrome of bronchiolitis, and this list is not exhaustive. Bronchiolitis (Tables 34-1 and 34-2) is most common during discrete seasonal outbreaks, and therefore an infant with bronchiolitis at the wrong time may warrant further evaluation. Similarly, recurrent or persistent bronchiolitis is a red flag as well. Bronchiolitis causes inflammation and damage within the bronchioles, with the resulting airway edema, excessive mucous production, and collection of cellular debris causing obstruction. This obstruction frequently leads to wheezing and respiratory distress and, therefore, can easily be mistaken for an asthma attack.

Table 34-1

Common Symptoms of Viral Bronchiolitis

- Fever
- Tachypnea
- Hypoxia
- Coryza
- Cough
- Wheezing
- Apnea in young infants

Table 34-2

Risk Factors for Severe Bronchiolitis

- Underlying conditions
  - Prematurity
  - Chronic cardiopulmonary disease
  - Immunodeficiency
- Epidemiologic factors
  - Passive smoke exposure
  - Lack of breast feeding
  - Birth from September through April
  - Multiple birth
  - Day-care attendance
  - Siblings

Bronchodilators have not been shown to have significant benefit overall for children with bronchiolitis[1]; however, there does seem to be a subset of these patients who do respond. Therefore, a trial of bronchodilators in the child younger than 2 years who presents with wheezing is a reasonable approach.

There are a number of less common causes of intrinsic airway obstruction that may present with wheezing and therefore mimic asthma. Recurrent pulmonary aspiration may cause chronic airway inflammation and edema. This may occur in infants with dysphagia (often associated with developmental delays), gastroesophageal reflux, or rarely an unrecognized H-type tracheo-esophageal fistula. Contrast swallowing studies are used to identify aspiration that may be causing wheezing in these cases. Other rare congenital structural abnormalities can lead to wheezing in infants. Among these are tracheal stenosis, tracheal webs, and tracheal hemangiomas (Figure 34-1). Patients with these lesions will frequently have stridor, but depending on the location of the lesion, these conditions may present with monophonic wheezing that does not respond to bronchodilators. Diagnosis is usually made by bronchoscopy. Cystic fibrosis is a genetic condition that affects the

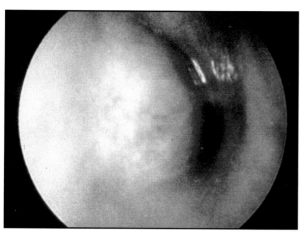

Figure 34-1. Image obtained at rigid bronchoscopy depicting an airway hemangioma resulting in near total obstruction of the mid-trachea. An obstructing lesion at this level may result in stridor, wheezing, or both.

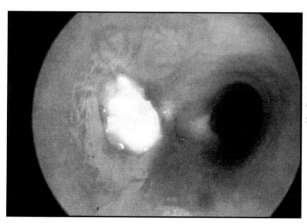

Figure 34-2. Image obtained at rigid bronchoscopy depicting an aspirated peanut obstructing the orifice of the left mainstem bronchus. Note the surrounding mucosal inflammation. Peanuts are notorious for ending up in the airways of young children due to their size, shape, and texture.

lung and airways that also may present as recurrent wheezing in a young child and should be considered especially in a child with failure to thrive or chronic diarrhea. Sweat testing should be performed to rule out this diagnosis. Congestive heart failure, whether due to unrecognized congenital heart disease or acquired disease, such as cardiomyopathy, may present with wheezing and respiratory distress due to pulmonary edema. Associated signs and symptoms, such as hepatomegaly, weak pulses, and dyspnea with feeding or activity, may be seen in these cases and may suggest this diagnosis. Local intrinsic airway obstruction may occur due to foreign-body aspiration (Figure 34-2). Bacterial infections such as bacterial tracheitis or even epiglottitis (Figure 34-3) can present with respiratory distress and noisy breathing that can be mistaken for asthma. Obviously, rapidly identifying the presence of these life-threatening emergencies is critical.

Extrinsic airway obstruction is a less common cause of wheezing in children. In the young child or infant, this may be caused by a vascular ring or sling. These occur due to congenital anomalies of the aortic arch that result in compression of the tracheobronchial tree and/or esophagus. Occasionally, these anomalies can be diagnosed on plain chest radiography if a right-sided aortic arch, significantly compressed trachea, or anteriorly bowing trachea is seen. Usually other imaging, such as contrast esophagram

Figure 34-3. Image obtained at rigid bronchoscopy depicting epiglottitis with severe inflammation and obstruction of the larynx.

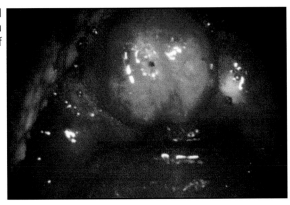

(looking for compression of the esophagus), CT, or MRI, is needed to make the diagnosis. Mediastinal lymphadenopathy or hilar lymphadenopathy due to conditions such as lymphoma, mycobacterial infection, or sarcoidosis can compress the airways and may cause wheezing. A large mediastinal tumor may also cause extrinsic airway obstruction and present with wheezing. A final important extrinsic cause of "wheezing" is not due to extrinsic compression of the airway, but due to vocal cord dysfunction. In patients with this condition, paradoxical vocal cord movement occurs with expiration, inspiration, or both. It can produce sounds of stridor or wheezing. In one type, the attacks seem to occur spontaneously, possibly due to panic or stress. In another, it occurs only with exercise and resolves with cessation of exercise.[2] The first type often occurs in patients who have asthma, so it can be a confusing picture. Often, these patients appear to be in significant distress, usually out of proportion to the degree of wheezing, and the pulse oximetry is normal. The diagnosis can be confirmed by direct visualization of the vocal cords with a nasal fiberoptic laryngoscope during an attack.

It is important to reiterate the truism that "all that wheezes is not asthma" when approaching a pediatric patient with acute airway symptoms. Similarly, the overlapping nature of physical findings, such as concurrent stridor and wheeze or simply noisy breathing, in young children can further cloud the picture. Following through on clinical clues and using targeted testing can often sort out the source of the symptoms.

References

1. Gadomski AM, Bhasale AL. Bronchodilators for bronchiolitis. *Cochrane Database Syst Rev.* 2006;3:CD001266.
2. Weinberger M, Abu-Hasan, M. Pseudo-asthma: when cough, wheezing, and dyspnea are not asthma. *Pediatrics.* 2007;120:855-864.

WHICH PATIENTS WITH ASTHMA IN THE EMERGENCY DEPARTMENT NEED TO BE ADMITTED TO THE HOSPITAL?

Jonathan E. Bennett, MD and Aaron S. Chidekel, MD

After a patient has been evaluated and treated for an asthma attack in the emergency department, a decision must be made on disposition: Is the patient safe to be discharged home, or should he or she be admitted to the hospital? An overview of the salient factors to consider is presented in Table 35-1, and while this list is certainly not meant to be exhaustive, it can guide a clinician's thinking. The patient's response to the initial therapy of bronchodilators and steroids largely determines the disposition, but other "nonmedical" factors play an important role as well and will be discussed below. Together, these clinical and nonclinical parameters create an impression of a patient who is either safe to be followed closely at home with ongoing outpatient medical therapy or who will require inpatient admission for more aggressive therapy and monitoring.

Those patients demonstrating a good response to the initial medical therapy as outlined in Questions 27 and 33 are candidates for discharge home on medical grounds. Children should show the return of good aeration of the lungs, and wheezing, if present, should be mild. Patients should have a good level of comfort and activity and demonstrate minimal signs of increased work of breathing. This constellation of clinical parameters should be maintained for approximately 1 to 2 hours after treatment. If this is the case, then the child is a candidate for discharge home with outpatient management and follow-up.

On the end of the spectrum, patients who do not respond to the initial medical therapy and who have persistently decreased aeration or have more than minimally increased work of breathing require admission to the hospital. Respiratory rate can be an important clinical parameter as well, particularly in young children. Age-specific normal values should be used, and the respiratory rate is best counted for a full minute and ideally when the child is in a quiet and afebrile state. Increasing respiratory rate has been shown to correlate with both increasing severity of airflow obstruction and decreased levels of

---

Table 35-1
Indications for Hospital and Intensive-Care Unit Admission

- Indications for hospital admission
  - Poor or incomplete response to initial therapy
  - Persistently increased work of breathing or tachypnea
  - Decreased oxygen saturation levels
  - Medical comorbidity that places the patient at increased risk
  - Psychosocial risk factors
  - Parental concern
- Consider intensive-care unit admission
  - Severe and persistent respiratory distress
  - Respiratory fatigue
  - Altered mental status
  - Poor air movement
  - Inadequate response to initial therapy
  - Medical comorbidity that places the patient at increased risk
  - Use of continuous inhaled bronchodilators

---

oxygenation. (This is true only in those patients who are not in imminent respiratory failure, as those patients may have slow respiratory rates, respiratory pauses, or even apnea due to exhaustion.) Additionally, patients with persistent hypoxia should be admitted to the hospital. While there is no specific cut point for oxygen saturation levels that can be set with certainty, lower oxygen saturation levels also correlate with increased levels of airway obstruction. Depending upon multiple factors, including the age of the child, the presence of co-morbid conditions, and the altitude above sea level, an oxygen saturation level between 92% and 94% breathing room air is a reasonable goal.

Patients with a clinical picture that falls in between these extremes and those who may respond transiently or incompletely and then either worsen or have a waxing and waning course require additional observation. This also provides the opportunity to obtain additional asthma history that can inform disposition, if not done already (Table 35-2). These children should continue on frequent (every 30 minutes to 1 hour) or even continuous nebulizer therapy with short-acting bronchodilators for an additional 1 to 2 hours. This may be done in an emergency department setting or, if available, in an observation unit. After this additional period of observation and treatment, those patients who respond and who can maintain this response off treatment for 1 to 2 hours can be discharged, while those failing the clinical test described above will require admission to the hospital.

Beyond clinical response, there are a few additional factors that might influence a decision to admit to the hospital or to discharge a child home from the emergency department. For example, if the child has already been on maximal therapy at home, has been using frequent bronchodilator therapy and oral corticosteroids, and does not have complete resolution of symptoms in the emergency department, admission should be considered. Additionally, if there is concern for the patient's ability to return easily to the emergency department should deterioration occur or if the parent feels uncomfortable with the child's condition and his or her own ability to provide ongoing asthma treatment, then

Table 35-2

Rapid Asthma Clinical History

- Prior medication usage
  - ○ Recent oral steroid usage
  - ○ Current oral steroid usage
  - ○ Steroid dependence
- History of previous exacerbations
  - ○ Rapid deterioration
  - ○ Emergency department visits
  - ○ Hospitalizations
  - ○ Intensive-care unit admission
  - ○ Episode(s) of respiratory failure
- History of current exacerbation
  - ○ Trigger
  - ○ Duration
  - ○ Comparative severity
- History of a significant medical comorbidity
  - ○ Underlying cardiopulmonary disease
  - ○ Extreme obesity
- Parental/family factors
  - ○ Parental assessment of severity or status
  - ○ Ability to care for child
  - ○ Transportation concerns
  - ○ Availability of outpatient medical follow-up
- Medication history
  - ○ Chronic outpatient medications
  - ○ Medications taken during this flare

the child should also be admitted. A significant comorbidity, particularly a concurrent cardiopulmonary diagnosis that may result in diminished respiratory reserve, will also tip the balance toward more conservative management and hospital admission. Finally, risk factors for a fatal asthma attack, as discussed in Question 32, should be considered when determining disposition, and if risk factors are present in a patient who does not have near complete resolution of symptoms, admission should also be considered.

Patients will occasionally be sick enough to require admission to an intensive-care unit. Those levels of therapies for patients with asthma that are supported in specific care environments will vary from institution to institution. For example, at my own hospital, we have the capability to provide continuously nebulized albuterol outside of the intensive-care unit. Similarly, the availability of continuous pulse oximetry and cardiorespiratory monitoring allows for closer monitoring of patients outside of the critical-care environment. With these caveats in mind, some clear medical indications for intensive-care unit admission include altered mental status or the impression of a high risk of respiratory failure or respiratory fatigue, poor air entry, the failure of the patient to improve despite aggressive initial therapy, and the prolonged need for continuous inhaled beta-agonist therapy. Some of the other factors that will point a patient toward an intensive-care unit include the history of previous intensive-care unit admission or respiratory failure or the presence of a significant medical comorbidity. Very high-risk medical comorbidities that have increased the likelihood of intensive-care unit admission include extreme obesity, significant bronchopulmonary dysplasia, myopathy, and significant underlying congenital heart disease.

The disposition of a patient with acute severe asthma or status asthmaticus is an important decision that involves medical and nonmedical parameters. A thorough history and clinical evaluation along with a conservative impression of the evolving disease process are all factors to consider. In general, the younger the child and the more severe the past history, the more conservative the decision about disposition will need to be to ensure patient safety. Geographic, socioeconomic, and cultural factors are important as well as is ensuring ongoing medical care and follow-up. Most patients with asthma will be safely discharged home from the emergency department and recover with ongoing outpatient therapy, but, due to the potentially life-threatening nature of pediatric asthma, it remains important to identify those children who really need to stay the night.

Suggested Readings

Chipps BE, Murphy KR. Assessment and management of acute asthma in children. *J Pediatr.* 2006;147:288-294.
Mannix R, Bachur R. Status asthmaticus in children. *Curr Opin Pediatr.* 2007;19:281-287.
Yock Corrales A, Soto-Martinez M, Starr M. Management of severe asthma in children. *Aust Fam Physician.* 2011;40:35-38.

WHAT IS THE STANDARD PRACTICE WHEN A PATIENT WITH AN ACUTE ASTHMA EXACERBATION IS ADMITTED TO THE HOSPITAL?

Lisa B. Zaoutis, MD

Hospitalization is warranted for patients with sustained or worsening respiratory distress during an asthma exacerbation or in patients where needed ongoing asthma therapy cannot reliably be continued after discharge. Continued or progressive asthma symptoms despite bronchodilator therapy is called status asthmaticus.

The goals of the hospital stay include the following:

- Management of status asthmaticus: Stabilization and improvement in asthma-related respiratory symptoms with appropriate escalation/de-escalation of respiratory support, treatments, and monitoring.

- Investigation and management of asthma triggers or comorbidities.

- Discharge planning (see Question 37):

    o Review of asthma history and home asthma care plan (postdischarge, maintenance, and acute exacerbation phases) with modifications made as needed.

    o Asthma education for patient and family.

    o Communication with primary or subspecialty medical team with appropriate postdischarge follow-up.

Standard Management of Status Asthmaticus

ASSESSMENT

Although a brief history and focused physical examination may be most appropriate when initially stabilizing a patient in respiratory distress, a complete history and physical examination should be completed as soon as possible because important co-morbidities may be revealed that could influence management. Chest radiography and laboratory studies are rarely needed in patients admitted with status asthmaticus. Exceptions include patients with persistent focal findings on auscultation, high fever or toxic appearance, severe chest pain, or other unusual clinical features.

The appropriate initial and ongoing assessment of the severity of the asthma exacerbation is essential. These assessments guide the type, amount, and frequency of treatments, as well as the trajectory of the course of illness.

Many institutions implement asthma pathways that link ongoing assessments and response to therapy to management. Patients are placed along a pathway according to their initial assessment and receive a corresponding therapy. As the patient demonstrates sustained improvement in severity of the asthma signs and symptoms, the intensity of the therapy and monitoring is reduced. When the patient reaches a level of therapy that can be maintained at home and demonstrates stability in his or her signs and symptoms on that home regimen, the patient is medically ready for discharge. Although asthma pathways may vary from one institution to another, a general sample is provided in Figure 36-1.

Most asthma pathways work well for the majority of patients without significant co-morbidities, but not for all patients with status asthmaticus. Some patients may tolerate a progression through the pathway at a faster rate, while other patients may require additional time or therapies to reach recovery. For some patients, worsening of their condition occurs despite appropriate treatment. In such cases or if the patient develops signs of respiratory failure (Table 36-1) or arrest, transfer to a facility or unit that can provide increased support (eg, intensive care unit) should be considered.

Medications

BETA AGONISTS

Inhaled short-acting beta-adrenergic agonists are the mainstay of hospital therapy. They stimulate beta-adrenergic receptors that cause relaxation of bronchial smooth muscle, which decreases airway obstruction. Other effects include stimulation of skeletal muscles (which can result in tremor), stimulation of cardiac muscles (which can cause tachycardia), and stabilization of mast cell membranes (which may decrease release of inflammatory mediators).

Albuterol is a commonly used short-acting selective beta-2-adrenergic agonist available for inhalation in a nebulizer solution or metered-dose inhaler (MDI). With a spacer and proper technique, albuterol administered by MDI is as effective as albuterol administered by nebulizer (Table 36-2). Levalbuterol is a preparation that offers the active R-enantiomer of albuterol and is dosed at half the milligram dose of albuterol.

Epinephrine is a nonselective adrenergic agonist and is most commonly used subcutaneously in patients who fail to respond to albuterol, especially in the early stabilization phase. Terbutaline is a selective beta-2-adrenergic agonist that can be used subcutaneously in place of epinephrine, but can also be administered as a continuous intravenous infusion for patients who deteriorate on inhaled beta-agonist therapy.

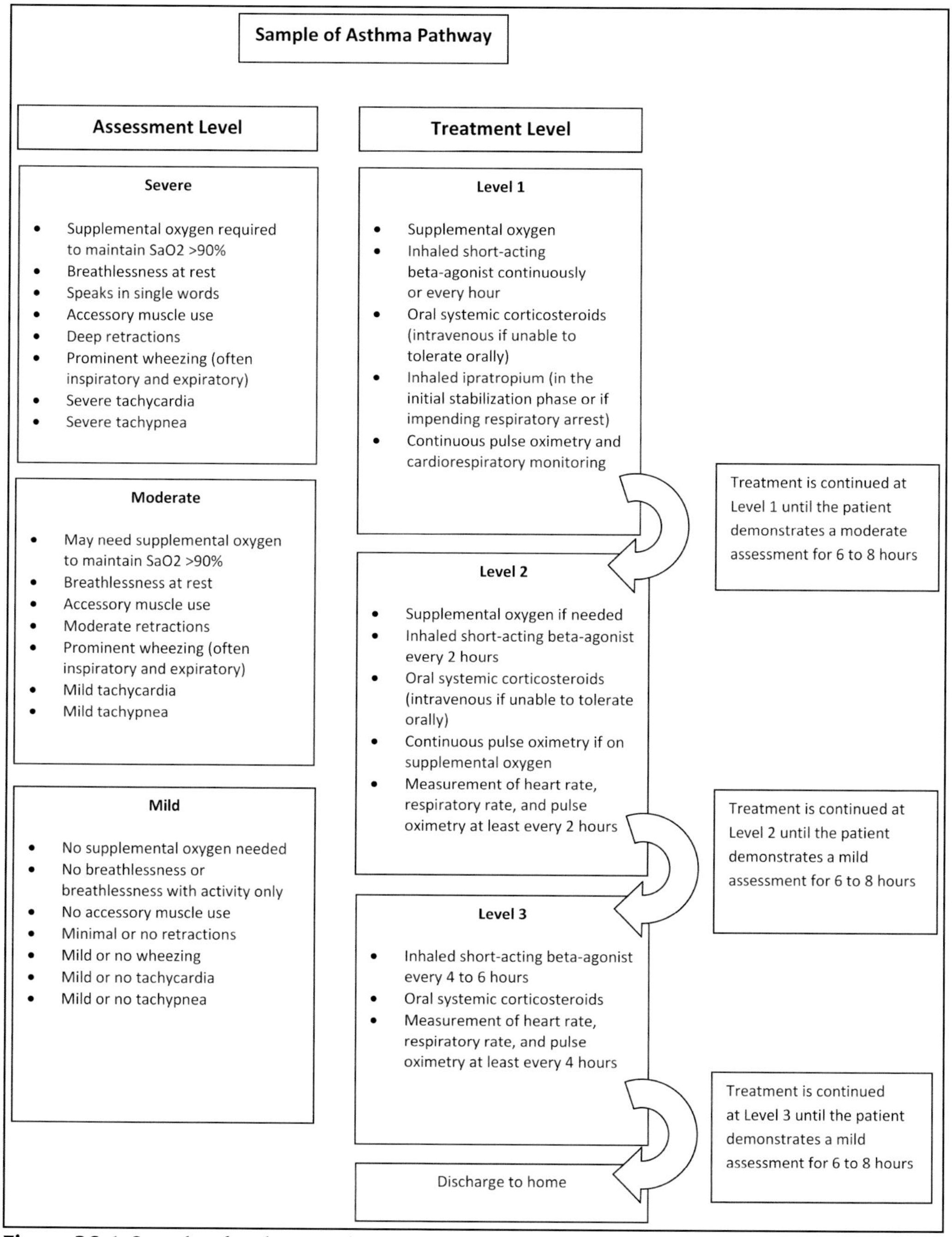

Sample of Asthma Pathway

Assessment Level	Treatment Level	
Severe • Supplemental oxygen required to maintain SaO2 >90% • Breathlessness at rest • Speaks in single words • Accessory muscle use • Deep retractions • Prominent wheezing (often inspiratory and expiratory) • Severe tachycardia • Severe tachypnea	**Level 1** • Supplemental oxygen • Inhaled short-acting beta-agonist continuously or every hour • Oral systemic corticosteroids (intravenous if unable to tolerate orally) • Inhaled ipratropium (in the initial stabilization phase or if impending respiratory arrest) • Continuous pulse oximetry and cardiorespiratory monitoring	Treatment is continued at Level 1 until the patient demonstrates a moderate assessment for 6 to 8 hours
Moderate • May need supplemental oxygen to maintain SaO2 >90% • Breathlessness at rest • Accessory muscle use • Moderate retractions • Prominent wheezing (often inspiratory and expiratory) • Mild tachycardia • Mild tachypnea	**Level 2** • Supplemental oxygen if needed • Inhaled short-acting beta-agonist every 2 hours • Oral systemic corticosteroids (intravenous if unable to tolerate orally) • Continuous pulse oximetry if on supplemental oxygen • Measurement of heart rate, respiratory rate, and pulse oximetry at least every 2 hours	Treatment is continued at Level 2 until the patient demonstrates a mild assessment for 6 to 8 hours
Mild • No supplemental oxygen needed • No breathlessness or breathlessness with activity only • No accessory muscle use • Minimal or no retractions • Mild or no wheezing • Mild or no tachycardia • Mild or no tachypnea	**Level 3** • Inhaled short-acting beta-agonist every 4 to 6 hours • Oral systemic corticosteroids • Measurement of heart rate, respiratory rate, and pulse oximetry at least every 4 hours	Treatment is continued at Level 3 until the patient demonstrates a mild assessment for 6 to 8 hours
	Discharge to home	

Figure 36-1. Sample of asthma pathway.

Table 36-1

Clinical Features of Impending Respiratory Failure

- Inability to speak
- Altered mental status (obtundation or extreme agitation)
- Poor air movement, rapid shallow breathing, decreased respiratory rate, or abnormal breathing motion
- Inability to lie supine

Table 36-2

Dosage of Standard Medication for Patients Hospitalized With Status Asthmaticus

	Route	*Dose*	*Frequency*	*Duration*
Albuterol nebulized solution	Inhaled	0.1 mg/kg (minimum 2.5 mg, maximum 10 mg)	Every 1 to 6 hours	Wean frequency of dosing during hospital stay until tolerating dosing no more frequent than every 4 to 6 hours.
Albuterol nebulized solution	Inhaled	0.5 mg/kg/ hour	Continuously	
Albuterol MDI (90 mcg/puff)	Inhaled	4 to 8 puffs	Every 1 to 6 hours	
Epinephrine 1:1,000	Subcutaneous	0.1 mg/kg (maximum 0.3 mg)	3 times every 20 minutes	
Prednisone or prednisolone	Oral	1 to 2 mg/kg/ day (maximum 60 mg/day)	2 divided doses/ day	Continue for 2 to 3 days after discharge (consider taper if longer than 2 weeks)
Methylprednisolone	Intravenous		4 divided doses/ day	

CORTICOSTEROIDS

Systemic corticosteroids are given routinely in hospitalized patients with an asthma exacerbation or status asthmaticus. Given early in the course of the exacerbation, it may prevent hospitalization, but, regardless, it is continued through the hospital stay to speed recovery and prevent recurrence. Prednisone or prednisolone given orally is standard. Methylprednisolone is the form for intravenous administration, but this is only needed in patients who cannot tolerate the medication orally (see Table 36-2).

INHALED ANTICHOLINERGICS

Ipratropium is the most commonly used inhaled anticholinergic bronchodilator. It is thought to provide additional bronchodilation by blocking cholingeric-mediated bronchoconstriction. Although it has been shown to reduce the rate of hospitalization when administered with albuterol in the emergency department, it has not been shown to provide additional benefit when continued in hospitalized patients.

SUPPLEMENTAL OXYGEN

Asthma produces changes in the lungs that include bronchospasm, airway edema, and increased mucous production, all of which can lead to atelectasis and mucous plugging. This can result in hypoxia, either episodic or more sustained. Supplemental oxygen, delivered through face mask with nebulized treatments or via nasal cannula, is warranted to maintain pulse oximetry levels above 90%. Transient desaturations that clear with cough, repositioning, or activity do not necessarily warrant supplemental oxygen therapy.

INTRAVENOUS FLUIDS AND ELECTROLYTES

Tachypnea and increased work of breathing can lead to inadequate hydration due to diminished oral intake and increased insensible losses. If encouraging oral intake of fluids is not successful, intravenous fluid supplementation may be warranted. Rehydration with intravenous normal saline if needed is an appropriate first step, followed by continuation of appropriate maintenance fluids (eg, D5-0.45NSS with 10 mEq/L potassium chloride) at a standard rate. Patients on continuous or frequent doses of inhaled beta-agonists can develop hypokalemia, so checking serum potassium levels is prudent, especially in patients requiring intravenous fluids.

NONSTANDARD THERAPIES

Additional treatments may be considered if symptoms worsen despite standard therapy. Depending on the expertise or experience of the clinicians or the support available in the setting, consultation with services that provide a higher level of care should be anticipated whenever possible.

Intravenous magnesium sulfate can be considered in patients with severe asthma exacerbations that fail to respond to intensive standard therapy. The desired effects include bronchodilation and mast cell membrane stabilization, but vasodilation can result in significant hypotension.

Heliox is a helium-oxygen gas blend that may improve ventilation and decrease work of breathing due to its lower density compared to air. Studies have been mixed in determining its efficacy in status asthmaticus, and it is often reserved for patients in impending respiratory failure. It has limited utility in patients with hypoxemia, and hypothermia has been an issue in some patients due to heliox's high thermal conductivity.

Therapies That Are Not Routinely Indicated in Status Asthmaticus

Certain therapies will have limited or no role in the routine management of status asthmaticus. Addition of medications and procedures that are not efficacious increase cost and complexity, and no therapy is completely risk free.

ANTIBIOTICS

Antibiotics should be reserved for use in those patients in whom there is clear evidence of bacterial infection. Realizing that the majority of episodes of status asthmaticus are triggered by viral infection, the presence of fever alone does not suggest the need to use antibiotic therapy.

COUGH SUPPRESSANT AND DECONGESTANT MEDICATIONS

Similar to antibiotics, the use of cough suppressant and decongestant medications is not indicated in the treatment of status asthmaticus.

CHEST PHYSIOTHERAPY

Chest physiotherapy is another therapy that is not routinely indicated in status asthmaticus. While mucous hypersecretion and even plugging of the airways is a component of asthma pathophysiology, there is no evidence that employing chest physiotherapy improves pulmonary function or length of stay. One potential exception to this statement is the occasional patient with status asthmaticus and lobar atelectasis who may benefit from more intensive airway clearance.

Differential Diagnosis

Alternative diagnoses should be considered in patients admitted for status asthmaticus, especially if they fail to respond to standard therapy or have an unusual presentation. A list of entities that can mimic asthma is listed in Table 36-3.

Summary

Status asthmaticus is a common reason for pediatric hospitalization. Its therapy is fairly standard and highly efficacious. Oxygen, inhaled bronchodilators, systemic corticosteroids, and clinical monitoring remain the foundation of inpatient therapy for pediatric status asthmaticus.

Table 36-3
Clinical Entities That Can Mimic Asthma

Entity	Salient Features
Anatomic airway abnormality	Frequent episodes of wheezing or cough in young infants or children that is often unresponsive to inhaled beta agonists
Inhaled foreign body	Unilateral symptoms in toddlers or older children with developmental delay
Gastroesophageal reflux	May be an alternative diagnosis or a contributory factor to asthma
Bronchiolitis	Wheezing accompanying or following upper respiratory illness in infants and children younger than the age of 2 years
Pneumonia, especially atypical (eg, *Mycoplasma, Chlamydia pneumoniae*)	Prominent rales, onset in a child with no previous wheezing history or family history of wheezing
Congestive heart failure	History of underlying heart disease, failure to thrive, murmur, hepatomegaly

Suggested Readings

Helzer M, Spergel JM. Asthma. In: Zaoutis LB, Chiang VW, Eds. *Comprehensive Pediatric Hospital Medicine.* Philadelphia, PA: Mosby Elsevier; 2007.

Johnson KB, Blaisdell CJ, Walker A, Eggleston P. Effectiveness of a clinical pathway for inpatient asthma management. *Pediatrics.* 2000;106:1006-1012.

Kercsmar CM. Acute inpatient care of status asthmaticus. *Respir Care Clin N Am.* 2000;6:155-170.

Schramm CM, Carroll CL. Advances in treating acute asthma exacerbations in children. *Curr Opin Pediatr.* 2009;21:326-332.

WHEN IS MY PATIENT WITH ASTHMA READY TO GO HOME?

Aaron S. Chidekel, MD

Because asthma remains the most common chronic disease of childhood and represents a very common but often preventable reason for hospital admission and emergency department visits among pediatric patients, discharge planning for and posthospital management of children with asthma will be a common scenario. Whether you are managing your own patients in the hospital, or whether they are managed by a hospitalist service that then hands that patient off to you for outpatient management, familiarity with asthma discharge criteria and planning and the initial posthospital management of children with asthma represents a critical component of safe and comprehensive asthma management.

Discharge planning for patients admitted to the hospital with an episode of status asthmaticus is multifactorial and multidisciplinary. It also begins at the time of admission. Most importantly, specific asthma-related and respiratory criteria for discharge must be met to ensure patient safety and a successful discharge home. In addition, as the prevention of hospital admission is a key goal of chronic asthma management, an inpatient hospitalization necessitates the re-assessment of the overall asthma care plan and the re-evaluation of the patient for previously unrecognized conditions (medical comorbidities) that may need to be treated. Importantly, a hospitalization can serve as a "teachable moment" to consolidate asthma teaching and the implementation of a more effective strategy for the future. At our institution, we focus on each of these elements when approaching the discharge for a patient admitted with asthma.

Some children with asthma experience recurrent exacerbations and require frequent hospitalization. These patients require particular attention and close follow-up. Recurrent hospitalization is a risk factor for a poor outcome or asthma death, and patients with frequent flares experience a high burden of disease. Anything that can be done to improve their health should be vigorously pursued.

Table 37-1

Asthma Discharge Checklist

- Medical issues
  - o   Acceptable level of comfort
  - o   No or minimal wheezing
  - o   Acceptable oxygenation breathing room air
  - o   Concurrent medical issues identified and controlled
  - o   Medical management in place
- Psychosocial issues
  - o   Environmental review
  - o   Access to medications and medical care assured
  - o   Primary provider for follow-up identified
- Educational issues
  - o   Asthma education
  - o   Written action plan provided
  - o   Contact information for medical care provided

From a medical standpoint, the discharge criteria for a patient with asthma are fairly straightforward (Table 37-1). A patient recovering from status asthmaticus is usually ready for discharge when albuterol treatments have been spaced to every 4 to 6 hours. Most often at our institution, we use a 4-hour interval as an acceptable criterion for discharge. The child should demonstrate favorable clinical parameters that can include an assessment of his or her overall level of comfort and work of breathing. We do not use specific asthma scores but rather rely on these factors as part of the overall clinical impression of how a patient is doing. Oxygenation as measured by pulse oximetry should be adequate while breathing room air, both awake and during sleep. While there is no agreed-upon magic number, most members of our group are comfortable with oxygen saturation values above 90% in an older child and above 92% in a younger child. (Our institution is at sea level.) Similarly, there is no agreement on the frequency of pulse oximetry measurements. This will vary from institution to institution. No matter what level of monitoring is the local practice at your hospital, it is most important to treat the patient and not the oximeter.

Auscultation of the chest should reveal good air exchange, and if wheezing is present, it should be minimal and improving. Findings that suggest pneumonia, atelectasis, or a diagnosis other than asthma should be recognized and addressed. Peak flow values may be used as an additional clinical parameter in the minority of patients in whom a peak flow-based action plan is available. Occasionally, spirometry can be obtained prior to discharge, but the value of this test may also be debatable during an asthma flare.

While a patient is in the hospital, any other comorbid medical conditions should be assessed and addressed, whether this is a previously recognized chronic problem or another new diagnosis. The hospitalization provides an opportunity to reassess the presence or absence of comorbid conditions and to facilitate any testing that may need to be performed. Most often, I recommend that testing be done as an outpatient and after a patient has returned to his or her baseline prior to performing new or important diagnostic studies.

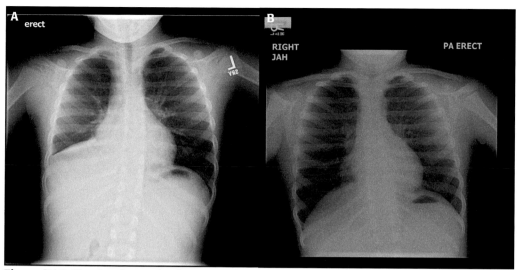

Figure 37-1. Chest radiographs demonstrating right lower lobe (RLL) collapse accompanying an asthma exacerbation. (A) RLL atelectasis. (B) Resolution of this finding. Atelectasis commonly accompanies status asthmaticus and may contribute to associated hypoxemia that precludes hospital discharge.

Similarly, any acute medical problems should be addressed, and, if not, resolving these should at least be controlled prior to discharge as well. This includes management of any intercurrent infection or other problem. If atelectasis is contributing to the severity of the asthma exacerbation (Figure 37-1), it should be recognized and a plan put into place for management and follow-up to ensure lung re-expansion. Similarly, any other exacerbating condition or newly recognized problem that will require ongoing therapy needs to be explained to the patient and parent so that management will be continued according to the medical needs of the child.

In addition to these medical parameters, attention is given to the other important aspects of asthma management prior to discharge as well. An assessment of the environment to which the child will be returning is undertaken. This focuses on exposure to environmental tobacco smoke and other asthma triggers, such as allergens in the home. Access to medications and medical care is ensured as well. Recent data suggest that many patients cannot afford their long-term controller medications, and the hospitalization enables the team to assess any additional resources that the family might need.

At our institution, respiratory therapists and nurses provide the patient and family with standardized and up-to-date asthma education. Online educational materials and videos are also accessible to patients and families. Some hospitals will have classes in asthma education given by certified asthma educators for families to participate in prior to discharge. Asthma education includes providing information about the pathophysiology of asthma and its many manifestations. Teaching about asthma triggers and comorbid conditions is provided as indicated. Education about medications and medication delivery systems and devices is provided as well. Finally, a written asthma action plan is prescribed by the medical team and provided to and reviewed with the patient and family prior to discharge. This is another common gap in management, and many patients with asthma report never being provided with a written action plan. There is plenty of time during a hospital stay to generate one! The overarching goal is to provide the patient and his or her family with the tools they need from medications to knowledge to get out of the hospital on the proper footing so as to avoid future hospitalizations.

After a hospitalization for an asthma flare, patients receive close follow-up in order to ensure safe transition to the home environment medically and to prevent a relapse of asthma symptoms and re-admission to the hospital. Preventing hospital re-admission is not only an important asthma quality outcome, but it is important to the safety and quality of life of the patient and his or her family as well. Most patients are discharged on increased medical therapies, such as oral corticosteroids; increased dosing frequencies of bronchodilators to control residual asthma symptoms; and often additional therapies for concurrent exacerbating conditions. Clinical follow-up is needed, as these therapies are tapered back to the patient's previous baseline asthma-care plan. Finally, follow-up is needed to ensure that the patient and his or her family have a good understanding of the overall asthma action plan moving forward.

Posthospital follow-up can occur in a number of settings. It is our practice to work collaboratively with primary-care physicians, allergists, and potentially other medical specialists to provide multidisciplinary care for the patients with asthma with whom we are involved. While we are the "medical home" for some of our asthma patients, the majority are followed primarily by their general pediatricians. No matter who is the main contact for the patient, it is important to identify the primary source of asthma follow-up as part of the discharge plan, and this is another potential gap in care that needs to be avoided.

In general, we maintain close contact with the patients with asthma for whom we will be serving as the primary point of contact. This is particularly the case for those who have more severe disease. Our inpatient nurse practitioner follows up directly by telephone with all patients discharged from our medical service within a week of hospital discharge. Patients are seen anywhere from 2 to 6 weeks after discharge by their primary pulmonologist, depending upon the specific needs of the patient and medical circumstances. This posthospital contact enables us to ensure a successful and safe discharge, to follow-up on or perform any testing, such as spirometry, or to gather any other information from the hospital stay, and to directly re-evaluate the patient to be sure that his or her asthma care plan is appropriate and sufficient.

Summary

Asthma discharge planning should be comprehensive, yet tailored to the needs of the individual patient. Medical parameters for discharge are generally straightforward. Rather, it is the complex integration of a chronic disease into the life of a child that often requires fine-tuning. Providing a clear and evidence-based medical regimen, a written asthma action plan, and targeted education will go a long way to prevent recurrent hospitalizations for your asthma patients, even those with severe disease.

Suggested Readings

1. Chidekel A, Marshall P. Acute asthma exacerbations roundtable. *J Asthma Allergy Educ.* 2010;1:71-74.
2. Helzer M, Spergel JM. Asthma. In: Zaotis LB, Chiang VW, eds. *Comprehensive Pediatric Hospital Medicine.* Philadelphia, PA: Mosby Elsevier; 2007.
3. Centers for Disease Control and Prevention. Vital signs: asthma prevalence, disease characteristics, and self-management education—United States 2001-2009. *MMWR.* 2011;60:1-7.

SECTION VII

ASTHMA EDUCATION

What Do Parents of My Patients Need to Know About Asthma and Its Management?

Concettina (Tina) Tolomeo, DNP, APRN, FNP-BC, AE-C

Parents should be informed about all aspects of asthma and its management at a basic level, but, most importantly, they need to understand that asthma is a chronic disease that can be controlled. Parents can gain this understanding if they realize the pivotal role inflammation plays in the disease process. It is this baseline knowledge that provides the foundation for understanding asthma symptoms, control, and therapy.

Unfortunately, many parents and children never receive or understand this important message. The Children and Asthma in America Survey, a telephone survey conducted between February and May 2004, revealed a widespread lack of understanding by children and parents about asthma causes, treatment, and symptom prevention. In this survey, the majority (93%) of respondents could not name inflammation as an underlying cause of asthma symptoms and thought (55%) it was only possible to treat asthma symptoms and not the underlying causes of asthma symptoms.[1] Other studies confirm that primary-care pediatricians do not routinely provide asthma education according to national guidelines. A recent study revealed that provision of asthma education during asthma-related visits significantly declined from 2001 to 2002 to 2005 to 2006.[2] In this study, age of 18 years or younger, receipt of long-term control medications, use of an allied health professional during the visit, and longer visit time were all independent predictors for providing asthma education. Asthma education was provided less frequently when patients with asthma had a non-asthma-related appointment.[2] To provide quality asthma care and management, all parents of children with asthma should receive information about asthma that will allow them to confidently and successfully self-manage their child's disease.

Asthma information should be provided at each encounter by each member of the health care team.[3] The information should be consistent across team members and should follow the recommendations put forth by the National Asthma Education and Prevention Program *Expert Panel Report 3*. Using pictures and models is an effective way

Figure 38-1. Airway model. Left: normal airway; Right: airway depicting inflammation and bronchoconstriction.

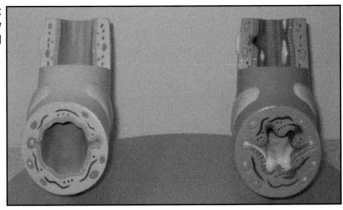

Figure 38-2. A visual aid for asthma severity. Onion ring: mild persistent asthma; chocolate donut: moderate persistent asthma; bagel: severe persistent asthma; cheese Danish: life-threatening asthma with mucous plugging. (Reprinted with permission from Zacharisen MC. A visual aid in asthma education. *J Asthma Allergy Educ.* 2010;1:77.)

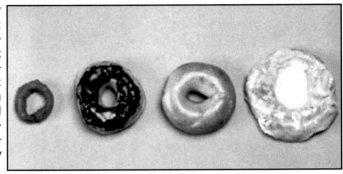

of communicating asthma information to both parents and children. Pictures and models can be elaborate, demonstrating what happens in the airways during an asthma attack (Figure 38-1); or they can be creative and simple, demonstrating the impact of inflammation on airway caliber (Figure 38-2).[4] Both examples allow you to further discuss the influence of environmental triggers on the inflammatory process as well as the purpose and importance of environmental control measures and medications. During this discussion, you should emphasize that controlling for environmental factors as well as adequate medication therapy are both critical components of asthma care and management.

Although the responsibility for the care and management of the child with asthma at home rests with the parents, more and more young children are assuming this role. In a study conducted to evaluate the association between child's age and controller medication responsibility, it was reported that, by age 7, a considerable number (almost 20%) of children assumed controller medication responsibility. This responsibility increased with age, demonstrating that, by age 11, about half of the children assumed responsibility, by age 15, most (75%) assumed responsibility, and by age 19, all (100%) assumed responsibility.[5] Thus, when providing information to parents, it is imperative that you not only include the child in the discussion early on in the disease process but that you provide the information at a level that is easily understood by both the parents and the child. It is important to engage the child in the conversation and not to assume that he or she is too young to be involved in the discussion of asthma management.

Even when this information is provided at a basic level, the sheer volume can be overwhelming. Therefore, at the first visit, it is vital that you make an assessment of the parents' and child's understanding of asthma, taking time to clarify any misconceptions. Once this has been accomplished, you must determine the minimum amount of information that can be conveyed to the parents at the first visit so that they can safely care for their child at home until the next office encounter. Often, this boils down to basic airway findings in someone with asthma, signs and symptoms of poorly controlled asthma and asthma exacerbations, the purpose and use of medications, when to call your office, and when to go to the emergency department. This is quite a lot in and of itself! At the follow-up visits, you can then focus on reviewing and reinforcing the information you provided at the first visit in addition to providing the parents and child with new information, such as environmental control measures.[3]

Summary

Parents and children should know the difference between a normal airway and the airway of a child with asthma, the airway changes that occur with asthma, and how to conduct an assessment of asthma control. Parents and children need to recognize and know what to do if symptoms are present. Understanding the difference between long-term controller and quick-relief medications and the importance of adherence to long-term controller medications is critical for implementation of and adherence to the medical plan. Finally, parents and children need to know about common environmental triggers and control measures.[3] Of course, the skills and education necessary to accompany these concepts are also essential and are discussed in Question 40.

References

1. *Children & Asthma in America, Executive Summary.* Research Triangle Park, NC: GlaxoSmithKline. GR1378R0. 2004.
2. Hersh AL, Orrell-Valente JK, Olson LM, Cabana MD. Decreasing frequency of asthma education in primary care. *J Asthma.* 2010;47:21-25.
3. National Asthma Education and Prevention Program. *Expert panel report 3 (EPR-3): guidelines for the diagnosis and management of asthma. Section 5: managing exacerbations of asthma.* Bethesda, MD: National Heart, Lung, and Blood Institute, 2007:373-417.
4. Zacharisen MC. A visual aid in asthma education. *J Asthma Allergy Educ.* 2010;1:77.
5. Orrell-Valente JK, Jarlsberg LG, Hill LG, Cabana MD. At what age do children start taking daily asthma medicines on their own? *Pediatrics.* 2008;122:e1186-e1192.

WHAT ARE SOME STRATEGIES TO ENHANCE ASTHMA EDUCATION IN MY PRACTICE?

Concettina (Tina) Tolomeo, DNP, APRN, FNP-BC, AE-C

Primary-care offices are typically very busy places. As a result, the educational needs of parents and children with asthma often go unmet.[1] Lack of time is a common reason reported for not providing asthma education in the primary-care setting.[2] However, providing asthma care consistent with the National Asthma Education and Prevention Program *Expert Panel Report 3* (NAEPP EPR-3) *Guidelines for the Diagnosis and Management of Asthma*, which includes self-management education, does not have to be time consuming. One study evaluated the effects on patients 2 years after pediatricians were taught by their peers to enhance their skills in asthma therapies and counseling. This study found that pediatricians who participated in the training benefited in important ways. Trained physicians received higher patient-rated performance scores regarding communication behaviors important to promoting patient's satisfaction and ability to manage asthma on their own, and in addition, their patients were also less likely to incur disruption of sleep caused by asthma symptoms. Another important finding of this study was that these positive results were achieved even though there was no difference in the time that peer-trained physicians spent with their asthma patients when first diagnosing a patient, seeing a new patient, or seeing a return patient. In fact, the peer-trained physicians spent less time with patients during urgent visits.[3] Such a method for enhancing education in your practice requires changing physician behavior.

System-level changes have also been evaluated. In one such study, researchers evaluated the effectiveness of 2 asthma-care improvement strategies in the primary-care setting. One was less time consuming and less expensive and consisted of peer leader education. The other was more intensive and more expensive and consisted of allocating a nurse to conduct planned asthma-care visits. This group also received peer education. Findings revealed that, although both strategies decreased asthma symptom days, the peer leader group did not reach statistical significance.[4] Therefore, when attempting to enhance

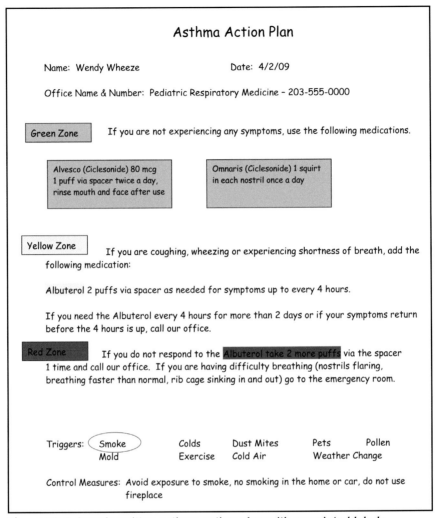

Figure 39-1. Sample written asthma action plan with preprinted labels.

educational practices in your office, it may be more effective to institute changes that target systems-oriented improvements, for example, developing a system that ensures all patients with asthma receive a written asthma action plan as per NAEPP EPR-3 Guidelines. One way to accomplish this is to automate the process by using an electronic medical record system. Such an approach makes it easy for the provider, legible for the patient and family, and a permanent part of the medical record. If instituting an electronic medical record is not feasible in your practice, having asthma action plans that are preprinted with medication names allowing you to check off or circle the treatment prescribed or having asthma action plans with a preprinted short-acting beta-agonist so that you only need to write the long-term control medications are 2 time-saving options. Creative shortcuts can also be useful. For example, color-coded labels for long-term control and quick-relief medications can be preprinted and then added to the action plan at the end of the visit. An example of such a plan can be found in Figure 39-1. All action plans described allow for individualization in an efficient manner.

Having written asthma action plans is only one step in the process for enhancing education in your office; using them is an even more important step. To encourage use of the action plans in your office, it is important to keep them readily available. Some suggestions include keeping the asthma action plans in each exam room so that they are easily accessible during each patient visit or having them clipped to the front of each asthma patient's chart before the visit begins.

Another method for enhancing education in your practice is to make resources available to your patients and to view each opportunity as a teachable moment. For example, providing patients and families with internet opportunities (such as the Quest for the Code asthma game found at www.asthma.starlight.org) for self-education while they are sitting in the waiting room or providing them with a list of resources (Table 39-1) that they can access at their convenience allows them to learn at their own pace. However, it is extremely vital to recognize that merely providing patients and families educational materials without providing explanation is not true education. All educational materials and resources provided to patients must be reviewed and reinforced by all members of your health care team. One way to accomplish this is to develop asthma-specific visit forms that include a list of key educational messages. This list can be used to prompt providers to introduce or review a message or messages at each visit. Thus, providing consistent and repeated educational messages by all members of your health care team is another step to enhancing education in your practice.

An alternative or supplementary method for providing self-management education and addressing key educational messages is to offer asthma education classes and resources in your office. Asthma education classes allow you to personally review important self-management concepts in a group setting, thus promoting efficiency as well as education. Numerous examples and forms (print, audio-video, online) of asthma educational resources are available that can also be tailored to meet the needs of an individual practice.

Two final recommendations for enhancing education in your practice include hiring a nationally certified asthma educator to provide education during patient visits as well as via telephone in between visits, and developing a system for referring patients who need additional education to asthma specialists. Both of these strategies are supported by the NAEPP EPR-3 Guidelines. The Guidelines recommend using health professionals and others trained in asthma self-management education to implement and teach asthma self-management. They also recommend referring patients who need additional education to improve adherence to asthma specialists.[5] National certification for asthma educators has been available since 2002; thus, it is relatively new, and the effectiveness of education provided by certified asthma educators has not been reported. However, numerous randomized controlled studies have reported improved asthma outcomes when patients and families were educated by someone specially trained in asthma care and self-management.[6]

Table 39-1

Asthma Education Resources for Providers and Families

Resource	*Phone Number*	*Web Site*
Allergy & Asthma Network Mothers of Asthmatics	1-800-878-4403	www.breatherville.org
American Academy of Allergy, Asthma, and Immunology	1-414-272-6071	www.aaaai.org
American College of Allergy, Asthma, and Immunology	1-847-427-1200	www.acaai.org
American Lung Association	1-202-785-3355	www.lung.org
Association of Asthma Educators	1-888-988-7747	www.asthmaeducators.org
Asthma and Allergy Foundation of America	1-800-727-8462	www.aafa.org
Centers for Disease Control and Prevention	1-800-232-4636	www.cdc.gov
National Heart, Lung, and Blood Institute	1-301-592-8573	www.nhlbi.org

---

Summary

There are many options for enhancing education in your practice; some are more labor-intensive and costly than others. Developing a system that fits within the confines of your practice makes quality asthma education accessible to all of your patients with asthma and their families, and using all members of your health care team is the best approach to enhancing asthma education in your practice.

References

1. McMullen A, Yoos HL, Anson E, Kitzmann H, Halterman JS, Sidora Arcoleo K. Asthma care of children in clinical practice: do parents report receiving appropriate education? *Pediatric Nursing.* 2007;33:37-44.
2. Peterson MW, Strommer-Pace L, Dayton C. Asthma patient education: current utilization in pulmonary training programs. *J Asthma.* 2001;38:261-267.
3. Clark NM, Cabana M, Kaciroti N, Gong M, Sleeman K. Long-term outcomes of physician peer teaching. *Clin Pediatr.* 2008;47:883-890.
4. Lozano P, Finkelstein JA, Carey VJ, et al. A multisite randomized trial of the effects of physician education and organizational change in chronic asthma care. *Arch Pediatr Adolesc Med.* 2004;158:875-883.
5. National Asthma Education and Prevention Program. *Expert panel report 3 (EPR-3): guidelines for the diagnosis and management of asthma. Section 5: managing exacerbations of asthma.* Bethesda, MD: National Heart, Lung, and Blood Institute, 2007:373-417.
6. Coffman JM, Cabana MD, Halpin HA, Yelin EH. Effects of asthma education on children's use of acute care services: a meta-analysis. *Pediatrics.* 2008;121:575-586.

What Education Should Be Provided to All Parents of Children With Asthma to Help With Day-to-Day Management?

Concettina (Tina) Tolomeo, DNP, APRN, FNP-BC, AE-C

Education is an integral component of the National Asthma Education and Prevention Program *Expert Panel Report 3* (NAEPP EPR-3) *Guidelines for the Diagnosis and Management of Asthma*. Asthma self-management education programs provided in a pediatric setting have been proven to be effective; however, the most important components of the educational interventions have not been identified.[1] The NAEPP EPR-3 Guidelines state that asthma education should include basic facts about asthma, assessing and defining asthma control, the role of asthma medications, instruction regarding inhaler and device technique, information about environmental triggers and control measures, instruction on how to self-monitor symptoms and/or peak flow rates, the provision of a written asthma action plan, how to handle signs and symptoms of worsening asthma, and information regarding when to seek medical care.[2] Table 40-1 lists details regarding the specific skills that should be included when providing asthma education to your parents, keeping in mind that the skills should be presented in a progressive fashion in order to avoid overwhelming the parents and child.

When providing information regarding the basic facts about asthma, you must be sure to speak at a level that the parents and child can understand. Using pictures and models can facilitate understanding. In addition, all education should be accompanied by written material that the parents and child can reference at home. This material should be written at no higher than the fifth-grade reading level and should be culturally appropriate.[2] When discussing medications, you should clearly explain the difference between long-term control and quick-relief medications. Correlating this information to the picture or the model can be useful. You must also explain to the parents and the child that long-term control medications do not work quickly and need to be used daily in order to be effective. This will help avoid the common pitfall of discontinuing long-term control medications before they have the opportunity to be effective. Providing anticipatory guidance

Table 40-1

Asthma Education Skills

- Role of inflammation in asthma
  - Differentiate between inflammation and bronchoconstriction
- Name, dose, schedule, purpose, refill recognition, priming, storing, and cleaning of medications (long-term control and quick relief) and devices
  - Explain difference between long-term control and quick-relief medications
- Inhaler (metered dose or dry powder) technique with/without spacer or holding chamber
  - Assess inspiratory flow rate as an objective measure
- Nebulizer technique—Including cleaning and storing equipment
- Self-monitoring skills utilizing symptom recognition and/or peak flow readings
  - Review common signs and symptoms
  - Determine patient-specific signs and symptoms
  - Instruction regarding peak flow zones
- Peak flow meter technique
- How to maintain symptom and/or peak flow diaries
  - Provide family with a symptom/peak flow diary
- How to read an asthma action plan
  - Provide plan in appropriate language
  - Explain what to do when well and when symptomatic
  - Provide plan that is culturally appropriate
- Trigger indentification and avoidance measures
  - Explain how to use a symptom diary to identify triggers
  - Provide personalized avoidance measures
  - Provide measures regarding where to obtain items such as an allergy-proof mattress and pillow covers
- Response to self-monitoring assessment
  - Explain what to do if signs and symptoms of worsening asthma are present
- Provide office telephone numbers for daytime and after-hour access

regarding this and other common pitfalls can help parents avoid these widespread practices. Common pitfalls to successful asthma self-management are provided in Table 40-2. Parents should also be instructed to ensure that the child has access to his or her short-acting beta-agonist at all times; this includes school and sporting activities. Furthermore, the importance of yearly influenza vaccination should be emphasized.

In addition to these basics of asthma, 2 other vital concepts are necessary for effective, quality asthma education: behavior modification and a partnership in care. Because asthma is a chronic disease, optimal control requires not only the use of appropriate medications, but the need for lifestyle changes. Therefore, in order for asthma education to be effective, it needs to include more than just the exchange of facts and information; it must incorporate behavior-modification techniques. Self-regulation is fundamental to behavior modification and includes self-assessment, judgment, and appropriate action.[3] Thus, asthma education should provide parents and children with the opportunity to learn and master these skills. One way to accomplish this is through the use of a written asthma action plan. After developing and reviewing the action plan with the parents and

Table 40-2

Successful Asthma Self-Management: Common Pitfalls By Topic, Cleaning

- Basic facts
  - o Lack of recognition of the role inflammation plays in asthma
- Medications
  - o Use of long-term control medications (prescribed as needed)
  - o Inappropriately discontinuing use of long-term control medications
  - o Overuse of short-acting beta-agonist
  - o Not having short-acting beta-agonist available at all times
  - o Inappropriate administration technique(s)
  - o Not using a spacer or holding chamber with metered-dose inhalers
  - o Inability to recognize the need for refills
  - o Improper priming and storing of medications
  - o Not cleaning inhalers and devices
- Environmental control measures
  - o Not clearning stuffed animals or favorite blanket on a regular basis
  - o Not washing bedding weekly in hot water
  - o Allowing smoking in one designated room of the home or apartment instead of allowing it outside the home and car
- Self-monitoring
  - o Misplacing written asthma action plan
  - o Not following written asthma action plan
  - o Not providing written asthma action plan to school
  - o Not calling when the action plan is not controlling/relieving symptoms
  - o Improper peak flow meter technique (ie, not forming a tight seal around mouthpiece or coughing into the peak flow meter)

the child, you should take the time to assess the parents' and child's understanding of the plan by asking, "What would you do if your child started to wheeze?" This question requires that the parents and child recognize that wheezing is a symptom of asthma, understand that the symptom requires an intervention, institute the intervention that consists of using a short-acting beta-agonist, and determine if the intervention was effective or not. Each stage along the way provides you with an opportunity to reinforce accurate steps and clarify those that were incorrect. The initial question can then be followed by, "What would you do if the wheezing continued or improved?" and "Show me how you would use the medicine." Fact-based questions such as, "What are the common symptoms of asthma?" and "What are the names of your medicines?" do not allow you to determine whether the parents and child have synthesized the information provided.

The second component of effective education is the development of a good working partnership with the parents and child. This can be accomplished by allowing for open communication, considering cultural and ethnic factors, identifying and addressing the parents' and child's concerns, identifying and addressing barriers to care, and developing mutual goals with the parents and child.[2] Such a relationship needs to be established early because a solid rapport with the provider and active parental and child participation can positively influence adherence and asthma control. Additionally, the concept of a partnership should expand beyond your office practice. To successfully manage asthma, you and your parents must partner with others who come in contact with or are involved in the child's care. This includes but is not limited to the child's teachers, coaches, pharmacists, and health insurance carrier. Working as a team is more effective than working alone.

References

1. Coffman JM, Cabana MD, Halpin HA, Yelin EH. Effects of asthma education on children's use of acute care services: a meta-analysis. *Pediatrics*. 2008;121:575-586.
2. National Asthma Education and Prevention Program. *Expert panel report 3 (EPR-3): guidelines for the diagnosis and management of asthma. Section 5: managing exacerbations of asthma.* Bethesda, MD: National Heart, Lung, and Blood Institute, 2007:373-417.
3. McGhan SL, Cicutto LC, Befus AD. Advances in development and evaluation of asthma education programs. *Curr Opin Pulmonary Med*. 2004;11:61-68.

SECTION VIII

ASTHMA TESTING

WHAT IS THE ROLE OF PULMONARY FUNCTION TESTING IN ASTHMA? WHAT TESTING SHOULD BE ORDERED AND WHEN?

Daniel J. Weiner, MD

Pulmonary function testing in asthma serves 2 main purposes: assisting in the initial diagnosis and monitoring asthma control (Table 41-1). The 2007 National Asthma Education and Prevention Program *Expert Panel Report 3* (NAEPP EPR-3): *Guidelines for the Diagnosis and Management of Asthma*[1] suggests that "spirometry measurements before and after bronchodilator should be undertaken for patients in whom the diagnosis of asthma is being considered." In this setting, spirometry can be used diagnostically by demonstrating obstructive disease that is reversible by bronchodilator. Obstructive disease that is not reversible (Figure 41-1), in the appropriate context, might suggest other diseases, such as bronchiolitis obliterans. Restrictive defects (Figure 41-2) might prompt further evaluation for chest wall, neuromuscular, or interstitial diseases. If baseline spirometry is normal and asthma is still suspected, provocative testing can be done. Inhalation of methacholine, mannitol, or cold, dry air have all been used to elicit bronchospasm and to determine the sensitivity of the airways. At the time of initial diagnosis, the degree of airflow abnormality helps in assessing asthma severity. Reduced FEV_1 or FEV_1/FVC ratio indicates current obstruction (impairment domain) and risk for future exacerbation (risk domain). For example, the impairment domain of the severity of asthma might be classified as mild ($FEV_1 > 80\%$ predicted), moderate (FEV_1 60% to 80% predicted), or severe ($FEV_1 < 60\%$ predicted).

Once the diagnosis of asthma is made, spirometry is also useful for assessing asthma control. One of the markers of "good control" is normal or near-normal lung function. The NAEPP EPR-3 recommends performing spirometry 1) at the time of initial assessment, 2) after treatment is initiated and symptoms and peak expiratory flow (PEF) have stabilized, 3) during periods of progressive or prolonged loss of asthma control, and 4) at least every 1 to 2 years thereafter. As a pulmonologist, I obtain spirometry at each follow-up visit (typically quarterly) and use this information to help determine whether increases or

Table 41-1

Pulmonary Function Tests Used in the Diagnosis and Monitoring of Asthma

Test	Uses	Advantages	Disadvantages
Spirometry	Measurement of airflow to assess airway caliber, responsiveness to bronchodilator or provocative agents.	Noninvasive. Reproducible. Technology relatively simple.	Requires time (15 min), experienced technician. Effort dependent.
Exhaled nitric oxide (eNO)	Measurement of eosinophilic airway inflammation.	Noninvasive. Requires less cooperation than spirometry.	Expensive technology ($6 to $8 per test). Not all asthma patients have elevated eNO. Measurement can be affected by diet.
Peak expiratory flow monitoring	Increased variability (day-to-day, morning to night) can indicate worsening asthma control.	Very inexpensive. Can be performed at home or school.	Insensitive to small airway obstruction. Less reproducible than spirometry and very dependent on effort. Does not indicate source of obstruction.

Figure 41-1. Flow volume curves before and after bronchodilator are very similar and both demonstrate concavity towards the volume axis. Note the relative preservation of peak expiratory flow (98% predicted) in comparison to other flow rates (FEV$_1$ 60% predicted, FEF$_{25-75}$ 32% predicted).

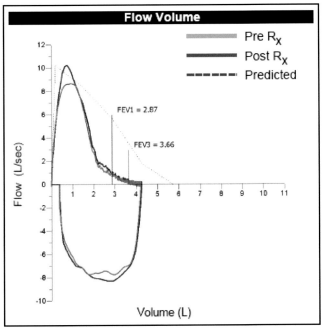

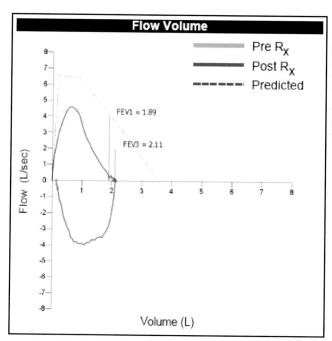

Figure 41-2. Flow volume curve from a patient with chest wall restriction due to radiation. The curve is quite narrow compared to the predicted (dotted) curve. The vital capacity is 60% of predicted and the total lung capacity is 68% predicted (measured by plethysmography, not shown).

decreases in medications may be warranted. This is clearly more often than is commonly measured in the primary-care setting. In a survey of 671 primary-care physicians (pediatricians and family physicians), a total of 429 physicians returned surveys relating to their practices regarding asthma care. Only 21% of respondents used spirometry routinely, and family physicians were nearly 6 times more likely than pediatricians to use spirometry in diagnosis.[2] Another more recent study reproduced these findings, suggesting that there remain significant barriers to the implementation of regular pulmonary function testing (spirometry) in primary-care settings. In this study, 52% of pediatricians and family practitioners used spirometry, but only 21% of primary-care physicians used spirometry regularly, and family practitioners were still more likely than pediatricians to use spirometry regularly.[3] However, another recent study demonstrated that prompts from an electronic medical record system were able to increase the utilization from spirometry, although the magnitude was small, the interpretation of the results is not described, and the impact on care was difficult to determine.[4]

PEF monitoring has also been used to monitor asthma control. An advantage of PEF is that the equipment is very inexpensive and that the test can be performed at home as often as requested. It should be noted that this measurement is highly effort-dependent, as is spirometry. However, spirometry usually provides several markers of adequacy of patient effort (eg, exhalation time, rapidity of rise of flow) that are not available with PEF. In addition, PEF reflects flows, primarily in the large airways, while spirometry provides measures of large airway and small airway flow; PEF may be relatively preserved despite severe small airway obstruction. The NAEPP EPR-3 Guidelines suggest that if home PEF monitoring is used, the patient's personal best peak flow should be used as the comparator. Additionally, long-term daily peak flow monitoring should be considered for patients who have moderate or severe persistent asthma, patients who have a history of severe exacerbations, and patients who poorly perceive airflow obstruction and worsening asthma. Patients in this last category can be particularly difficult to treat and may progress from "well" outpatients to the intensive care unit within hours.

The NAEPP EPR-3 also recommends objective measurements of lung function (FEV_1 or PEFR) during acute exacerbations to help judge the severity of the exacerbation. As the patient improves, these same measures can help determine readiness for discharge. The NAEPP EPR-3 Guidelines state that "discharge is appropriate if FEV_1 or PEF has returned to ≥70% of predicted or personal best and symptoms are minimal or absent."[1] Although not specifically addressed in the guidelines, I find spirometry at discharge helpful to guide the duration of systemic steroid therapy. A patient who is very close to his or her baseline lung function may do well with a shorter course, while patients more than 20% from their baseline lung function may need longer (or tapering) courses of steroids.

Increases in the fraction of exhaled nitric oxide (FeNO) are thought to reflect the intensity of eosinophilic airway inflammation. Elevated FeNO may predict responsiveness to inhaled corticosteroids. One prospective, controlled study showed that when inhaled corticosteroids (ICS) treatment was adjusted to control FeNO, as opposed to controlling the standard indices of asthma, the cumulative dose of ICS was reduced, with no worsening of the frequency of asthma exacerbations.[5] However, the magnitude of ICS dose reduction was fairly small. In my practice, I have not found FeNO useful for making or refuting a diagnosis of asthma, which highlights that there are a variety of asthma phenotypes, not all of which have eosinophilic inflammation.[6] I have found it very useful for monitoring disease activity in a subset of patients who have elevated FeNO.

Other lung function tests (eg, measurement of lung volumes or diffusing capacity) may be helpful to exclude other diagnoses, but do not contribute significantly to the evaluation of patients with a straightforward history consistent with asthma.

References

1. National Asthma Education and Prevention Program. *Expert panel report 3 (EPR-3): guidelines for the diagnosis and management of asthma*. Bethesda, MD: National Heart, Lung, and Blood Institute, 2007. NIH publication no. 08-4051.
2. Finkelstein JA, Lozano P, Shulruff R, et al. Self-reported physician practices for children with asthma: are national guidelines followed? *Pediatrics*. 2000;106(4 Suppl):886-896.
3. Dombkowski KJ, Hassan F, Wasilevich EA, Clark SJ. Spirometry use among pediatric primary care physicians. *Pediatrics*. 2010;126:682-687.
4. Bell LM, Grundmeier R, Localio R, et al. Electronic health record-based decision support to improve asthma care: a cluster-randomized trial. *Pediatrics*. 2010;125:e770-e777.
5. Smith AD. Use of exhaled nitric oxide measurements to guide treatment in chronic asthma. *N Engl J Med*. 2005;352:2163-2173. Epub 2005 May 24.
6. Fajt ML, Wenzel SE. Asthma phenotypes in adults and clinical implications. *Expert Rev Respir Med*. 2009;3:607-625.

Is Office-Based Spirometry Possible? How Do I Interpret the Results?

Daniel J. Weiner, MD

Office-based spirometry is indeed possible, but not necessarily easy. The resources required are a cooperative patient, proper equipment, and experienced staff with adequate time. Most children over the age of 6 can perform spirometry, and there is good evidence that a substantial portion of 4- to 5-year-old children can as well. Younger or less cooperative patients may require more time to test. A number of manufacturers make spirometry equipment that is laptop-based and suitable for office use. Some manufacturers use disposable flow sensors, which may have some potential for erroneous results.[1] Others use traditional differential pressure pneumotachs with disposable mouthpieces/filters. These devices can be obtained for $1500 to $2500.

Probably more important than the equipment, however, is having staff trained in coaching the patient to properly perform spirometry. Spirometry requires the patient to take a maximal inhalation followed by a maximal and prolonged exhalation. Submaximal efforts can give very inaccurate results, underestimating some parameters (vital capacity, forced expiratory volume in one second), while potentially overestimating others (forced expiratory flow between 25% and 75% of vital capacity, FEF_{25-75}). Testing sessions also require that these difficult maneuvers be performed several times and demonstrate reproducibility. This can require a great deal of patience on the part of the staff, who must also be able to work with children of different ages. A healthy, cooperative patient might be able to perform an acceptable test in approximately 10 to 15 minutes, but a distractible patient performing the test for the first time might require 30 minutes. If the pediatrician wished to assess responsiveness to a bronchodilator (Figure 42-1), this requires the ability to administer bronchodilator (2 minutes by metered-dose inhaler, and 10 minutes by nebulizer), wait 15 minutes for bronchodilator effect, and then repeat spirometry (an additional 10 to 15 minutes). This time requirement may be difficult to accommodate in a busy office setting when routine visits themselves may be only 10 to 15 minutes long.

Figure 42-1. Flow volume curve before (green) and after (red) bronchodilator, demonstrating significant bronchodilator response. Pre-bronchodilator FEV$_1$ 74% predicted, FEV$_1$/FVC ratio 58%, FEF$_{25\text{-}75}$ 36% of predicted. Post-bronchodilator FEV$_1$ 118% predicted (23% increase), FEV$_1$ 92% predicted, FEF$_{25\text{-}75}$ 49% predicted (36% increase). These results are consistent with but not diagnostic for asthma.

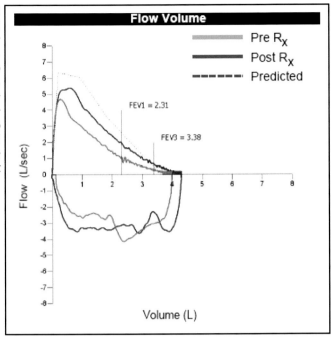

Additionally, technician coaching is improved with regular experience. If spirometry is performed infrequently and irregularly, it is difficult to maintain good test quality.

The feasibility of performing office spirometry has been examined in both adult and pediatric populations. In one study, 10 pediatric practices were each provided with 10 hours of didactic and hands-on instruction and were expected to perform at least 30 spirometries over 12 weeks.[2] Feedback on the test quality was provided by pediatric pulmonologists. Thereafter, 109 children underwent spirometry both in the office setting and the hospital PFT laboratory. The good news is that 78% of the office tests were considered acceptable by American Thoracic Society criteria. The bad news was that 21% of studies were not interpreted correctly by the pediatricians. One of the conclusions of this study was that an integrated approach, involving both the primary-care center and the pulmonologist, is important to ensure quality results. The National Asthma Education and Prevention Program *Expert Panel 3* recommends that "when office spirometry shows severe abnormalities, or if questions arise regarding test accuracy or interpretation, further assessment should be performed in a specialized pulmonary function laboratory."[3]

Many spirometry software systems will provide a computerized interpretation of the results. I have found that these interpretations perform better for tests in adults than in children and perform poorly if the test quality itself is suboptimal. It is critical that pediatric reference equations be used by the computer when testing children; inappropriate use of adult equations can provide very misleading results. There are several excellent resources for learning about spirometry performance and interpretation,[4,5] but doing this well also requires doing it frequently. If you choose to undertake office spirometry, consider exploring whether your local pediatric pulmonologist is able to assist with interpreting study results.

References

1. Townsend MC, Hankinson JL, Lindesmith LA, Slivka WA, Stiver G, Ayres GT. Is my lung function really that good? Flow-type spirometer problems that elevate test results. *Chest.* 2004;125:1902-1909.
2. Zancanato S, Meneghelli G, Braga R, Zacchello F, Baraldi E. Office spirometry in primary care pediatrics: a pilot study. *Pediatrics.* 2005;116:792-797.
3. National Asthma Education and Prevention Program. *Expert panel report 3 (EPR-3): guidelines for the diagnosis and management of asthma.* Bethesda, MD: National Heart, Lung, and Blood Institute, 2007. NIH publication no. 08-4051.
4. *Spirometry fundamentals.* University of Washington Interactive Medical Training Resources, Seattle, WA. Retrieved from www.depts.washington.edu/imtr/spirotrain/programs/spirofun/index.html.
5. Quanjer P. *Become an expert in spirometry.* Retrieved from www.spirxpert.com/.

WHAT OTHER TESTS WILL MY PATIENT WITH ASTHMA NEED?

Natalie M. Hayes, DO

This question considers 2 common scenarios in pediatric practice. The first situation involves the patient with chronic respiratory symptoms that are consistent with asthma and in whom the diagnosis needs confirmation and comorbidities assessed. The second scenario involves the ongoing follow-up of a patient with chronic asthma in whom periodic assessment and monitoring is required to be consistent with guideline-based asthma care as well as the evaluation for comorbidities should difficulties in asthma control arise. Because asthma is such a common clinical problem in pediatric practice, it is in the best interest of both the patient as well as the practitioner if a standard testing approach to or philosophy about asthma and its common comorbidities is employed. This is by no means suggesting that every patient with possible asthma be given a "rubber-stamp" evaluation, but rather that the practitioner making the assessment knows which tests to order at the appropriate time to aid in the diagnosis and management of the individual patient.

Testing will be needed based on other comorbidities that your patient may have or need to have ruled out. History and physical examination are the critical determinants of which testing will be needed and how urgently they may need to be obtained. Any red flags in the history, such as a history of severe symptoms or respiratory failure, a history suggestive of atopy or anaphylaxis, or a history of frequent infections, will suggest certain tests. As discussed below, allergy testing and immunologic testing are commonly obtained at some point in the evaluation and management of a child with asthma. Similarly, any physical examination features that are concerning or atypical for asthma will also require a prompt and thorough evaluation. Failure to thrive, clubbing, and crackles in a preschool-aged child will demand a different testing strategy than new-onset focal wheezing in an adolescent, yet both require prompt and appropriate evaluation if the diagnosis of cystic fibrosis is to be made in the first case and new-onset Hodgkin's lymphoma in the second (Figure 43-1). The history and physical examination of the patient with respiratory

Figure 43-1. Mediastinal masses are uncommon but important causes of new-onset or atypical wheezing in children and adolescents. Intrathoracic airway compression from the expanding tumor mass results in airflow obstruction and wheezing. Airway obstruction may become life-threatening. In this case, Hodgkin's lymphoma resulted in new-onset wheezing in a 12-year-old patient.

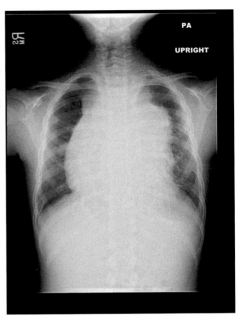

symptoms is critical to track common problems and to pick up the occasional rare condition that is masquerading as asthma. However, because these things are common in medicine, testing for the patient with either established asthma or newly considered asthma is most often straightforward and non-urgent. Spirometry and chest x-ray are the most commonly obtained tests in patients with asthma and are discussed in more detail elsewhere.

Suffice it to say that spirometry is critical in the confirmation of airway obstruction, documenting its reversibility and severity and evaluating bronchial hyper-reactivity. Spirometry should be obtained regularly in any patient who is taking chronic medications for asthma so that management may be stepped up or down in accordance with the patient's level of lung function and symptom control. Peak flow values alone are not sufficient to monitor pulmonary function in childhood asthma. School-aged patients can often perform accurate spirometry, but there will be some variability in the ability of individual patients, and some selectivity may be required. Any physician managing patients with asthma should identify a venue where their patients with asthma can have their lung function measured efficiently and accurately, whether this is right in your own office or in the pulmonary function testing (PFT) laboratory of the local hospital. If the local hospital is not a children's hospital, a quick phone call to the PFT lab will confirm that the hospital does indeed test children and of what age. Other tests of lung function, such as lung volume measurements and lung diffusion, are less important in the ongoing management of asthma than is spirometry. Occasionally, a patient with asthma will require pulmonary challenge testing as part of his or her evaluation. Cardiopulmonary exercise testing can quantify the patient's response to exercise and can help to clarify the complaints of exercise intolerance and chest pain or to assess the role of exercise-induced bronchospasm. Exercise testing can be done with concurrent flexible laryngoscopy to assess vocal cord motion during exercise when there is a question of vocal cord dysfunction. Other challenge testing may include isocapnic cold air or methacholine challenge testing to evaluate bronchial hyper-reactivity.

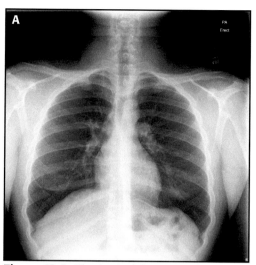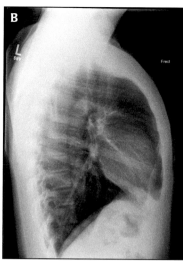

Figure 43-2. The typical features of asthma are well-depicted on this chest radiograph of an adolescent with persistent asthma. In the AP view (A), peribronchial thickening is evident as is evidence of hyperinflation of the lungs. Hyperinflation is often best seen on the lateral chest radiograph (B) with flattening of the diaphragms and expansion of the retrocardiac air space.

Radiographic studies should be tailored to the clinical question at hand. If a previous chest x-ray has been completed, any follow-up studies should address a specific question rather than be done for screening purposes. The initial chest x-ray may be normal or may demonstrate common features of asthma (Figure 43-2). Additional radiographic studies may be required from time to time. Possible scenarios include sinus imaging in patients with chronic sinus disease that is complicating asthma management and lateral neck films in patients with chronic congestion, mouth breathing, or middle ear disease.

Cystic fibrosis (CF) is the most common life-shortening genetic disease in Whites. CF occurs in people of all races, however, and often presents with chronic respiratory symptoms that may be similar to asthma. Common respiratory symptoms include cough, chest congestion, with or without wheezing, and recurrent upper and lower respiratory tract infections. CF is a multisystem disease, however, and nonrespiratory complaints, particularly gastrointestinal complaints, are also common. While all 50 states now have newborn screening in place for CF, any patient with a truly chronic cough (particularly a chronic wet cough) should have a sweat test. Associated failure to thrive or persistent crackles makes this recommendation more urgent than routine. The sweat test should be done at an accredited CF care center to reduce the occurrence of either false-positive or false-negative results. Additionally, patients with clubbing, nasal polyps, or rectal prolapse also warrant a sweat test in a timely fashion. Genetic testing is also available for CF, but sweat chloride testing remains the gold standard first-line test.

Many patients with asthma also have an allergic component. This may present as allergic rhinitis, eczema, or even food allergy. The presence of food allergy is an additional risk factor for more severe asthma. While antihistamines or intranasal steroids can be trialed to control allergic symptoms, if symptoms are uncontrolled, further testing can be helpful. An elevated serum immunoglobulin-E (IgE) level or eosinophilia from a complete blood

---

Table 43-1

Red Flags for Potential Immunodeficiency

- More frequent infection than expected
  - Recurrent bacterial pneumonia
  - Frequent otitis media in an older child
  - Persistent sinus or ear disease
- More severe infection than expected
  - Recurrent invasive bacterial disease
  - Invasive bacterial infections in multiple sites
- Frequent infections despite the lack of an epidemiological risk factor
  - Day care attendance
  - Multiple siblings
  - Tobacco smoke exposure
- Opportunistic infections
- Poor growth
- Features suggestive of an underlying syndrome or diagnosis

Adapted from Lederman HM, Gelfand EW. Approach to the child with recurrent infections. In Leung DYM, Sampson HA, Geha RS, Szefler SJ, eds. *Pediatric Allergy: Principles and Practice*. St. Louis, MO; Mosby: 2003.

---

count can nonspecifically indicate an allergic disposition and correlate with risk of asthma persistence. An extremely high IgE requires further evaluation as it may suggest allergic bronchopulmonary aspergillosis or simply severe atopy. Radio-allergosorbent (RAST) testing and/or allergy skin prick testing can identify specific substances to which a patient is allergic. RAST testing is done on a blood sample, and many potential allergic triggers can be tested. Skin testing is a procedure that is performed in the physician's (most often an allergist's) office. While the results of allergy testing may not correlate perfectly with the clinical response of the patient, identifying potential triggers in an objective fashion with testing can certainly guide environmental control. In young children, allergy testing may be less reliable as the immune system may not be fully developed.

A patient with recurrent upper or lower respiratory tract infections may require an initial workup for immunodeficiency with serum immunoglobulins. This should be considered in patients with frequent illnesses, particularly in young children (Table 43-1). While significant immunodeficiency usually presents with recurrent invasive bacterial infections in more than one site (bacterial pneumonia and meningitis, for example) or unusual infections (such as fungal disease or *Pneumocystis carinii* pneumonia), it is not at all uncommon to order these studies. It is important to be aware of the development of the immune system and use age-specific normal values for immunoglobulin levels. Specific antibody titers to vaccines such as tetanus or pneumococcus can be ordered as well, as part of a more detailed evaluation. Thankfully, severe immunodeficiency disorders such as severe combined immunodeficiency and Wiskott-Aldrich syndrome are quite rare.

Evaluation of the "aerodigestive system" is often indicated in young children with chronic respiratory symptoms and asthma. Airway films, including airway fluoroscopy, can evaluate for tracheobronchomalacia, and an upper gastrointestinal series (UGI) is helpful in determining whether a vascular ring or sling may be present. Together, these studies provide a noninvasive means of detecting overt anatomic abnormalities in the airway. However, if there is adequate suspicion, further testing with either bronchoscopy or more detailed imaging may still need to be undertaken, and some patients with complex problems will require multiple studies to enable an adequate understanding of their airway anatomy and physiology. Gastroesophageal reflux is a commonly considered asthma comorbidity. If reflux is noted during the upper GI study, then this study is helpful with diagnosing reflux. However, a negative upper GI study cannot rule out reflux, as an episode may not occur during the study. This is also true for a gastric emptying scan, which may document reflux more easily because the study evolves over a more prolonged period of time. A pH study or a dual multichannel intraluminal impedance-pH monitoring is another test that is available to document reflux. With dual multichannel intraluminal impedance-pH monitoring, all reflux events are documented, both acidic and nonacidic. According to Pilic and colleagues,[1] of 700 measurements using both pH and multichannel intraluminal impedance monitoring in patients ranging from age 3 weeks to 16 years, 270 measurements were abnormal, with 120 of the events abnormal only from impedance monitoring. In this study, 320 subjects tested had pulmonary symptoms. Additionally, 133 of the 320 subjects had abnormal values, and 77 of these (58%) were with impedance monitoring only. If indicated, upper GI endoscopy can be performed to evaluate for reflux or eosinophilic esophagitis.

If primary ciliary dyskinesia is suspected, due to recurrent sino-pulmonary infections or due to the presence of situs inversus, a tracheal or nasal brushing or biopsy should be obtained. The sample is examined under electron microscopy to determine whether ultrastructural abnormalities of the cilia are present. Olin and colleagues recently described an outpatient technique for obtaining a nasal scrape biopsy.[2] With this technique, 88% of the samples were able to be interpreted out of 448 specimens from 107 young children (range: 0 to 5 years), 189 older children (range: 5 to 18 years), and 152 adults (older than 18 years).

Vocal cord dysfunction may co-exist with asthma as well. This condition commonly masquerades as difficult-to-treat asthma or exercise-induced asthma. It is a condition that can be difficult to diagnose, but it may be suspected when there is flattening of the inspiratory loop during spirometry. Nasolaryngoscopy may need to be performed to diagnose paradoxical vocal fold motion, and this may also be performed as part of an exercise study in the appropriate setting. Patients with vocal cord dysfunction may benefit from speech therapy to learn breathing exercises to help control future episodes.

Summary

The evaluation of a patient with asthma may need to be comprehensive if symptoms are severe and involve more than one organ system. Conversely, in a well-appearing child with typical asthma symptoms and a more benign history and physical examination, spirometry and chest radiography may be all that are required. Patients with established asthma should have regular evaluation with spirometry, and other testing should be considered if evidence of a new comorbidity arises. Testing should be sensible and streamlined to eliminate unnecessary cost and procedures, and testing should be specific to the clinical question at hand. Every patient with asthma does not need every single test, rather he or she needs those results that will guide the therapy that will contribute to the best possible outcomes.

References

1. Pilic D, Fröhlich T, Nöh F, et al. Detection of gastroesophageal reflux in children using combined multichannel intraluminal impedance and pH measurement: data from the German Pediatric Impedance Group [published online ahead of print October 28, 2010]. *J Pediatr.* doi:10.1155/2011/271404.
2. Olin JT, Burns K, Carson JL, et al. Diagnostic yield of nasal scrape biopsies in primary ciliary dyskinesia: a multicenter experience [published online ahead of print January 31, 2011]. *Pediatr Pulmonol.* doi: 10.1002/ppul.21402.

Suggested Reading

Heinle R, Linton A, Chidekel A. Exercise-induced vocal cord dysfunction presenting as asthma in pediatric patients: toxicity of inappropriate inhaled corticosteroids and the role of exercise laryngoscopy. *Ped Asthma Allergy Immunol.* 2003;16:215-225.
Lederman HM, Gelfand EW. Approach to the child with recurrent infections. In: Leung DYM, Sampson HA, Geha RS, Szefler SJ, eds. *Pediatric Allergy: Principles and Practice.* St. Louis, MO: Mosby; 2003.

SECTION IX

OTHER MANAGEMENT PEARLS

Why Is the Influenza Vaccine so Important for the Patient Diagnosed With Asthma and What Other Vaccines Do My Patients Need?

Joel D. Klein, MD, FAAP and Jennifer LeComte, DO

All pediatric patients and practitioners should adhere to the immunization schedule recommended by the American Academy of Pediatrics (AAP) and the Advisory Committee on Immunization Practices (ACIP). The AAP recommends annual trivalent seasonal influenza immunization for all children and adolescents 6 months of age and older. This recommendation is further delineated to focus on the protection of people at higher risk for influenza-related complications and emphasizes that patients with chronic pulmonary conditions, including those with asthma, receive the influenza vaccine. Patients diagnosed with asthma are a priority group even when vaccine supply is limited.

The AAP purposefully recommends the trivalent seasonal influenza immunization (TIV), a killed vaccine, for all patients younger than 2 years old and for those who carry a diagnosis of asthma. A live-attenuated influenza vaccine (LAIV) is administered intranasally for healthy people aged 2 to 49 years. The LAIV is not recommended for those with a history of wheezing. Studies have shown that medically significant wheezing was observed more frequently in children younger than 24 months of age after vaccination with the LAIV. To further define at-risk patients, the AAP recommends asking parents/guardians of children ages 2 to 5 the following question: "In the previous 12 months, has a health care professional ever told you that your child had wheezing?" A positive response is a contraindication to using the LAIV. This recommendation is based on the pre-licensure studies that identified a possible association between LAIV and episodes of wheezing among children younger than 5 years of age.

Influenza remains an important cause of hospitalization and outpatient visits among all young children. This burden of illness is even greater among patients with asthma. The influenza vaccine is important because health care utilization rates are higher among children with asthma and influenza infection when compared to healthy children with influenza. In one study, children 6 to 59 months of age with asthma had about 4-fold more influenza-attributable hospitalizations and 2-fold more outpatient visits than did healthy children. Ironically, the asthma group in this study also had a 3- to 4-fold increase in parental reporting that their child received vaccination against influenza.

Vaccination rates for children with asthma unfortunately have remained low (less than 30%) despite the specific recommendations for vaccination by the AAP and ACIP. It is unclear why vaccination rates remain so low. One theory is that health care providers defer vaccination because of concern about the efficacy and safety of influenza vaccination, especially during asthma exacerbations. This clinical question is often a concern because the availability of the annual influenza vaccine and the peak of asthma season coincide in the fall. Another reason for low vaccination rates against influenza may be concern that the vaccine could result in an asthma exacerbation. Several studies have indicated that there is no significant increase in asthma exacerbations immediately following the administration of the inactivated influenza vaccine. Another study specifically addressed the administration of the TIV during an acute asthma exacerbation and concurrent use of prednisone. Park and colleagues studied the safety and immunogenicity of influenza vaccination during an acute asthma exacerbation and specifically included patients with asthma on steroid therapy and found that antibody response to influenza in the prednisone-treated and control groups were not different.[1] Adverse effects, including asthma exacerbation, were also no different between the 2 groups. The Committee on Infectious Diseases of the AAP recommends deferral of influenza immunization in patients receiving high-dose steroids, equivalent to prednisone 2 mg/kg, but the deferral should be temporary and should not compromise the likelihood of eventual immunization. However, this recommendation may result in missed opportunities for immunization.

Bacterial infections that result in respiratory illnesses may be more severe in children with asthma. *Streptococcus pneumoniae* can cause pneumonia and can result in symptoms of fever, cough, shortness of breath, and chest pain. Pneumococcal vaccination is currently included in the schedule of routine immunizations recommended by the AAP and ACIP. At the present time, asthma is not a specific indication for Pneumovax, unlike some other chronic pulmonary and immunologic conditions. Despite this, some asthma specialists recommend and administer this vaccine to patients with asthma, and this is not unreasonable. Pneumococcal vaccination remains an area that is evolving in terms of vaccines that are available and specific indications. *Haemophilus influenzae* type b (Hib) is a severe bacterial infection that can result in pneumonia, and its transmission is most likely through respiratory droplets. Hib vaccination is currently included in the schedule of routine immunizations recommended by the AAP and ACIP. Pertussis, a respiratory illness commonly known as whooping cough, is a very contagious disease caused by *Bordetella pertussis*. It is usually spread by coughing or sneezing while in close contact with others, who then breathe in the pertussis bacteria. Pertussis vaccination is also currently included in the schedule of routine immunizations recommended by the AAP and ACIP. Recent outbreaks and deaths from pertussis emphasize the importance of this safe and efficacious vaccine, and adolescents and pregnant women are particularly important groups in whom to ensure adequate protection. While infections with *Streptococcus pneumoniae*, *Haemophilus influenzae*, or *Bordetella pertussis* have not been noted to occur more frequently in patients with asthma, vaccine-induced protection against respiratory infections would likely benefit patients diagnosed with asthma in addition to the influenza vaccine.

In a Cochrane review in 2008, there was no firm evidence from a controlled clinical trial to support universal vaccination against influenza among patients with asthma. However, more recent data did show that asthma quality-of-life scores may be improved with the administration of the influenza vaccine. Even with mixed evidence, it is my practice to recommend the influenza vaccine to all patients diagnosed with asthma and extend the recommendation to their family members in order to minimize transmission to a vulnerable asthmatic patient. The recently updated recommendations for universal influenza vaccination of all children aged 6 months and older reinforces this important concept. Finally, adherence to the other components of the immunization schedule also benefits the asthmatic patient.

References

1. Miller EK, Griffin KM, Edwards KM, et al. Influenza burden for children with asthma. *Pediatrics*. 2008;121:1-8.

Suggested Readings

Cates CJ, Jefferson TO, Rowe BH. Vaccines for preventing influenza in people with asthma. *Cochrane Database Syst Rev*. 2008;2:CD000364.
Centers for Disease Control and Prevention. Prevention and control of influenza with vaccines—recommendations of the Advisory Committee on immunization practices (ACIP) 2010. *MMWR*. 2010;59(RR08):1-62.
Park CL, Frank AL, Sullivan M, Jindal P, Baxter BD. Influenza vaccination of children during acute asthma exacerbation and concurrent prednisone therapy. *Pediatrics*. 1996;98:196-200.

WHAT IS THE ROLE OF THE UPPER AIRWAY IN ASTHMA AND HOW BIG OF A PROBLEM IS SINUSITIS AND ALLERGIC RHINITIS?

Stephen J. McGeady, MD

The observation that individuals with bronchial asthma often have disease of the upper airway has led to inquiry into the possible connection between the 2 areas. The concept that these areas do have a connection, such that disease in one can affect the other, is known as integrated airway disease or one airway hypothesis or sometimes as united airways disease. There are several lines of evidence supporting a connection between disease of the upper and lower airways, and evidence will be considered under the headings Observational, Physiologic, and Pharmacologic.

Observational Evidence

Observational evidence of a connection between asthma and disease of the upper airway has been found in a number of reports. Among children with allergic rhinitis, a prevalence of asthma of up to 40% has been reported[1] compared to approximately 7% in the general pediatric population. If the association is considered conversely, the prevalence of allergic rhinitis among patients with asthma has been found to be as high as 90% even when rigorous criteria for allergic rhinitis are applied.[2] This greatly exceeds the prevalence of allergic rhinitis in the general population, which is 10% to 20%.[3] Further evidence of a connection was found in a longitudinal study of 690 college freshmen who had no evidence of asthma. A 23-year follow-up found that those who reported symptoms of allergic rhinitis as freshmen were almost 3 times as likely to have asthma (10.5%) as those who had no nasal symptoms (3.6%).[4] A commonly observed phenomenon among asthmatic patients is found in the above study in that the onset of allergic rhinitis symptoms precedes those of asthma. This sequence was also noted in a report of 13- to 17-year-old children who had both rhinitis and asthma: 59% either experienced nasal symptoms first or both diseases appeared in the same year.[5] These studies suggest that upper airway diseases may predict the development of asthma and infer a close connection. The above-referenced studies note the frequent association of rhinitis and asthma; however, a similar increase of sinus disease has also been reported among asthmatics. Studies in recent years have shown that between 40% and 60% of patients with asthma also have abnormalities on sinus radiographs.[1] In one report, patients with asthma considered moderate or severe had more sinus symptoms and greater abnormality on CT scans of the sinuses than individuals with mild asthma, suggesting that the severity of sinus disease may influence that of asthma or vice versa.[6]

Physiologic Observations

Physiologic observations of the connection between disease of the upper airway and bronchial asthma have led to the proposal of a number of possible causes of this association.

- Naso-bronchial reflex. Although the literature has not been consistent in accepting such a connection, the presence of a naso-bronchial reflex has been postulated to explain the finding of subjects experiencing an immediate increase in airway resistance when irritating stimuli are applied to the nasal mucosa.[7] Other investigators have failed to demonstrate a change in airway resistance, but have found that challenge of the nasal mucosa with allergen in ragweed-allergic subjects produced an increase in airway responsiveness to methacholine inhalation.[8] Both of these phenomena might be explained by naso-bronchial reflex, but, as noted, some studies have failed to confirm the evidence of such a reflex.

- Systemic allergic inflammatory response is a term referring to the hypothesis that an allergic reaction occurring in the nose or sinuses might produce systemic effects by generation of cytokines and chemical mediators. The existence of this mechanism has been suggested by increased bronchial hyper-reactivity following nasal allergen challenge as noted above, but also by the converse finding of increased numbers of eosinophils in the nasal mucosa when a segmental endobronchial allergen challenge is carried out in allergic subjects.[9]

- Mouth breathing due to nasal obstruction has been proposed to cause asthma by decreasing the nasal passages' effect of warming and humidifying inspired air because inspiration of cold and dry air has been shown to be a cause of bronchospasm.[10] The nasal function of removing particulates from inspired air also minimizes the exposure of the lungs to allergens and pollutants. These nasal functions are lost when the individual with severe rhinitis and/or sinusitis breathes through the mouth, and asthma may be aggravated as a result.

- Postnasal drip of secretions due to nasal and/or sinus inflammation has been suspected as a cause of increased asthmatic changes in the bronchi. Studies to determine whether nasal secretions actually enter the lower airways, however, have not been consistently positive. Some show that secretions may be aspirated,[11] while others fail to demonstrate aspiration.[12] This mechanism must be considered unproven, although physiologically plausible.

Pharmacologic Evidence

Pharmacologic evidence convincingly shows that effective treatment of rhinitis and sinusitis has a beneficial effect on asthma symptoms. This benefit has been shown both for antihistamine therapy and for intranasal glucocorticoids. Consideration of the benefits of antihistamine therapy in asthmatics is complicated by the fact that histamine H1 receptor antagonists have been shown to have a direct beneficial effect on lung function.[13] Thus, observed improvement in asthma when these drugs are given to patients with both allergic rhinitis and asthma cannot be ascribed solely to their effects on upper airway disease, although rhinitis is improved by the therapy. A number of studies have shown improvement in asthma symptoms following antihistamine introduction, although a concomitant improvement in objective markers of asthma severity has not been consistently demonstrated.[8] Studies of the effect of intranasal glucocorticoids on asthma symptoms are more straightforward to interpret because it has been demonstrated that only trivial amounts of the intranasal steroid reaches the lower airway, and the direct steroid effects can be assumed to be limited to their effect on the upper airway. One particularly impressive study found asthmatic symptoms to be greatly reduced by use of intranasal steroids but not by cromolyn or placebo.[14] A retrospective study evaluated 13,800 patients in a managed-care organization, and both children and adults were tracked for 3 years. Patients who received nasal steroids have a 30% lower risk of asthmatic flares requiring emergency department care compared to asthmatics not receiving such therapy.[15]

When taken together, the results of observational studies, reports of evidence of the physiologic connections between disease of the upper and lower airways, and the findings of studies of the effects of the therapeutic interventions strongly support the existence of an integrated airway in which disease of the nose or sinuses can affect the course of bronchial asthma. Clinicians who treat patients with asthma can expect better clinical outcomes if they are aware of this connection and apply therapies to both the upper and lower airways when appropriate.

References

1. de Benedictis FM, del Giudice MM, Severini S, Bonifazi F. Rhinitis, sinusitis and asthma: one linked airway disease. *Paediatr Respir Rev.* 2001;2:358-364.
2. Kapsali F, Horowitz E, Fogias A. Rhinitis is ubiquitous in allergic asthmatics. *J Allergy Clin Immunol.* 1999;99:S138.
3. Pedersen PA, Weeke ER. Allergic rhinitis in the same patients. *Allergy.* 1983;38:25-29.
4. Settipane RJ, Hagy GW, Settipane GA. Long-term risk factors for developing asthma and allergic rhinitis: a 23-year follow-up study of college students. *Allergy Proc.* 1994;15:21-25.
5. Van Arsdel PP Jr, Motulsky AG. Frequency and hereditability of asthma and allergic rhinitis in college students. *Acta Genet Stat Med.* 1959;9:101-114.
6. Bresciani M, Paradis L, Des Roches A, et al. Rhinosinusitis in severe asthma. *J Allergy Clin Immunol.* 2001;107:73-80.
7. Kaufman J, Wright GW. The effect of nasal and nasopharyngeal irritation on airway resistance in man. *Am Rev Respir Dis.* 1969;100:626-630.
8. Corren J. Allergic rhinitis and asthma: how important is the link? *J Allergy Clin Immunol.* 1997;99:S781-S786.
9. Braunstahl GJ, Kleinjan A, Overbeek SE, Prins JB, Hoogsteden HC, Fokkens WJ. Segmental bronchial provocation induces nasal inflammation in allergic rhinitis patients. *Am J Respir Crit Care Med.* 2000;161:2051-2057.
10. Griffin MP, McFadden ER Jr, Ingram RH Jr. Airway cooling in asthmatic and nonasthmatic subjects during nasal and oral breathing. *J Allergy Clin Immunol.* 1982;69:354-359.

11. Huxley EJ, Viroslav J, Gray WR, Pierce AK. Pharyngeal aspiration in normal adults and patients with depressed consciousness. *Am J Med.* 1978;64:564-568.
12. Bardin PG, Van Heerden BB, Joubert JR. Absence of pulmonary aspiration of sinus contents in patients with asthma and sinusitis. *J Allergy Clin Immunol.* 1990;86:82-88.
13. Bousquet J, Godard P, Michel FB. Antihistamines in the treatment of asthma. *Eur Respir J.* 1992;5:1137-1142.
14. Welsh PW, Stricker WE, Chu CP, et al. Efficacy of beclomethasone nasal solution, flunisolide, and cromolyn in relieving symptoms of ragweed allergy. *Mayo Clin Proc.* 1987;62:125-134.
15. Adams RJ, Fuhlbrigge AL, Finkelstein JA, Weiss ST. Intranasal steroids and the risk of emergency department visits for asthma. *J Allergy Clin Immunol.* 2002;109:636-642.

HOW MANY CHEST X-RAYS ARE ENOUGH? WHEN SHOULD I ORDER IMAGING STUDIES, AND WHICH STUDIES SHOULD BE DONE?

Julie Ryu, MD

Every test has its risks as well as its benefits. I would only order a test if the results would change my clinical decision or management, and the same is true for x-ray studies. It is usually more common to order imaging studies during the initial evaluation of a patient with chronic respiratory symptoms, but once a diagnosis is established and treatment initiated, it is best to order studies much more selectively and based upon clinical changes or questions that come up. Personally, I think one chest x-ray is enough unless clinically indicated.

Chest x-rays are a great screening tool for respiratory disorders but they have their limitations. Some common indications for ordering a chest x-ray are 1) a first-time wheezing episode, 2) a positive tuberculosis skin test (PPD), 3) focal breath sounds are heard, 4) pneumonia is suspected, 5) increased work of breathing or low oxygen saturations, and/or 6) during the evaluation of a patient with a history of a chronic cough (Figure 46-1). These are just some general indications when to order a chest x-ray. I typically do not repeat a chest x-ray in a patient with documented asthma unless pneumonia or a new pathologic process is suspected. Although the increased risk of cancer is extremely low with a single chest x-ray, the risks are cumulative, and therefore even a chest x-ray should be ordered judiciously to minimize any long-term risks. Chest x-rays are helpful but are often insufficient as a sole diagnostic tool.

Chest computed tomography (CT) is an excellent tool to investigate the lung parenchyma because it allows for a cross-sectional image of the chest. Chest CT can be very helpful in diagnosing lung disorders, such as interstitial lung disease, pneumonia with or without empyema, bronchiolitis obliterans, bronchiectasis, lung masses, congenital lung disorders, and airway abnormalities. Chest CT with contrast should be ordered to visualize vascular structures to determine if a lung mass is vascularized or to visualize lymph nodes as in a patient suspected of having hilar adenopathy. Contrast is also helpful in determining

Figure 46-1. This is a chest radiograph from a 14-month-old girl with a 3-week history of cough, revealing a triangular density in the right hilar region and subtle air trapping (hyperlucency) in the right lower lobe. Rigid bronchoscopy with retrieval of a piece of glass from the right mainstem bronchus was performed and resulted in resolution of her symptoms.

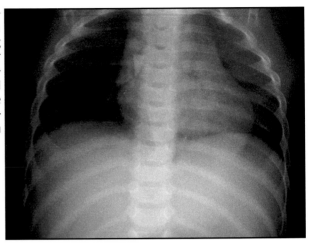

Figure 46-2. Contrast-enhanced chest computed tomography image revealing a double aortic arch in a 3-year-old boy undergoing evaluation for chronic cough and wheeze, which had been persistent since early infancy. As part of his initial evaluation, a chest radiograph and barium swallow were performed, and these revealed a right-sided aortic arch. An MRI can also be performed to define vascular anatomy.

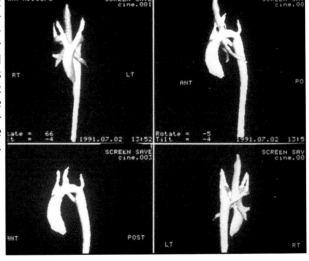

if there is vascular compression of airways (Figure 46-2) or to determine if pulmonary lesions are calcified. While rare in pediatrics, a chest CT with contrast should be ordered when pulmonary embolism is suspected.

In addition to the cross-sectional views that a CT can provide, many centers are able to create 3D images, making visualization of the chest much more accessible to the nonradiologist. Three-dimensional images are a great way for the nonradiologist to visualize complicated anatomy. The CT can also be used not only diagnostically, but also therapeutically. CT-guided procedures can be helpful in the removal of loculated fluid in empyema or when performing a biopsy of a lesion. Overall, the chest CT is an easily accessible and very helpful diagnostic tool. However, a chest CT results in much higher doses of radiation exposure than a chest x-ray and therefore should be ordered judiciously as well.

Airway fluoroscopy can be a useful tool in diagnosing airway pathologies. The advantages of airway fluoroscopy are that it requires no sedation, is quick, and can assess airway patency in real time. Thus, it is often used to diagnose laryngo- or tracheomalacia because the airway may appear normal on exhalation but narrows on inspiration.

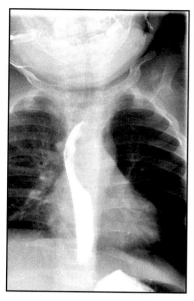

Figure 46-3. Barium esophagram image obtained in a 12-month-old boy evaluated for chronic wheezing, revealing esophageal deviation due to the presence of a large bronchogenic cyst.

Functional abnormalities such as malacia may be missed or under- or over-estimated on a single capture point as on CT but likely to be better evaluated on airway fluoroscopy because this test can visualize the airway dynamically.

Barium esophagram/upper gastrointestinal series (UGI) can be a useful tool to evaluate vascular structures in cases where a vascular ring is suspected. Similarly, if the esophagus is compromised due to the presence of a mediastinal mass (Figure 46-3), it will be detected as well. In addition, an UGI may provide some insight into the presence of gastroesophageal reflux, although other studies can also evaluate for this common condition. If there is a question about swallowing function, the barium swallow can be performed in the presence of a speech pathologist as well.

Flexible bronchoscopy can be a diagnostic as well as a therapeutic tool. It is often used to collect broncho-alveolar lavage (BAL) fluid to identify an organism during an infection. Pediatric pulmonologists perform flexible bronchoscopy as opposed to rigid bronchoscopy, which is usually performed by an otolaryngologist. The benefit of flexible bronchoscopy is the ability to reach the lower airways and the right upper lobe, which can sometimes be difficult to access with a rigid scope. Therefore, flexible bronchoscopy allows fluid to be obtained from a particular segment of the lung. In addition, the risk of pneumothorax and bleeding is much lower than that of a rigid scope due to the inherent malleability of a flexible bronchoscope.

Common studies performed on BAL samples include cell count, which may help identify certain disorders such as collagen vascular disease, or cancers, which alter the normal cellular ratio of neutrophils and lymphocytes. Macrophages can also be stained for lipid or hemosiderin. Lipid-laden macrophages are often present with chronic microaspiration, and hemosiderin is found in patients with hemoptysis or pulmonary bleeding. BAL fluid can also be gram-stained and cultured for bacteria, viruses, and fungi. Although cultures can always be sent, if the patient is receiving antibiotics, the probability of identifying a bacterial organism lowers with time.

Chest magnetic resonance imaging (MRI) is rarely ordered in pediatric respiratory disorders. Currently, the MRI of the chest does not image the lung parenchyma well. However, it is an excellent imaging tool to visualize vasculature and does not use any ionizing radiation as does CT and chest x-ray, but uses magnetic fields to create an image. While the advantages of MRI consist of no radiation, the time required for imaging is extensive and usually requires sedation.

Ultrasonography of the chest is a useful diagnostic tool that is not associated with any radiation. It can be used to distinguish chest wall masses from cystic lesions, to distinguish fluid collection from pneumonia on a "white out" on chest x-ray, and to follow effusions. In addition, ultrasound can be useful in detecting diaphragm abnormalities. Ultrasound of the diaphragm can measure diaphragm thickness during contraction and therefore may be a good tool to assess patients with diaphragmatic dysfunction.

Suggested Readings

Brenner DJ, Hall EJ. Computed tomography—an increasing source of radiation exposure. *N Engl J Med*. 2007;357: 2277-2284.

Frush DP, Donnelly LF, Chotas HG. Contemporary pediatric thoracic imaging. *AJR Am J Roentgenol*. 2000;175: 841-851.

How Can I Maximize Patient Adherence to Therapy?

Concettina (Tina) Tolomeo, DNP, APRN, FNP-BC, AE-C

The issue of adherence to therapy is complicated and multifactorial. Improving adherence in your practice begins with recognizing that nonadherence is a widespread problem and realizing there are numerous reasons for nonadherence. These 2 steps will help you identify and appropriately address nonadherence in your patient population.

It has been repeatedly reported that adherence to therapy is low in both children and adults and reaches its nadir during the adolescent years.[1] Unfortunately, nonadherence is often not identified by providers and results in an increase in asthma symptoms and resource utilization. Asking a simple question, such as, "How often do you miss your medicines?" will help open the lines of communication. Asking the question in a non-threatening manner gives parents and children the impetus needed to admit their medication-taking habits and reveal their reasons for nonadherence and barriers to adherence.

Numerous reasons for nonadherence have been reported. They can be categorized as patient related, caregiver related, or disease/treatment related. Examples of patient-related factors include psychological disorders, lack of insurance, and alternative health beliefs. Examples of caregiver-related factors include long wait times, inconvenient office hours, and lack of communication. Disease- or treatment-related factors include medication side effects, the need for prophylactic therapy, and the chronic nature of the disease.[2] Forgetfulness is the primary reason identified for nonadherence. A recent review of qualitative studies of adherence revealed the following reasons for nonadherence as identified by children with asthma and their parents:

- Not wanting to be viewed as different by other children.
- Fear of side effects.
- Fear of dependence on inhaled steroids.
- Difficulty experienced by parents when administering medications; this was partly due to resistance from the child.

- Challenges associated with coordinating the sharing of responsibility for treatment among children and caregivers, including other family members, teachers, and babysitters.[3]

All reasons can be classified into 2 broad categories—volitional and inadvertent. Volitional nonadherence occurs when the parent or child makes a conscious decision to not take medications as prescribed based on his or her knowledge and/or perception of disease severity and/or treatment benefits. As a result, they purposefully cut back, miss, or alter doses to match their need. For example, parents may feel that the risks associated with daily inhaled corticosteroid therapy outweigh the benefits of their effectiveness and thus choose to not give their child the medication. Inadvertent nonadherence occurs when someone fails to follow a treatment plan because of barriers. For example, parents may not understand the difference between long-term control and quick-relief medications and, thus, may administer the long-term control medication to their child on an as-needed basis instead of daily.[2]

Because of the different variables associated with each category of nonadherence, interventions aimed at maximizing adherence to therapy must be geared toward meeting the needs of the individual child and family. This is usually best accomplished by using a combination of strategies to encourage adherence. Furthermore, because asthma is a chronic disease managed by instituting daily medications and lifestyle changes, assessment and promotion of adherence must go beyond medications, it should encompass all components of self-management including, but not limited to, spacer/holding chamber use, trigger control and avoidance, and attendance at regularly scheduled appointments.

A recent study of children with asthma used focus groups to further describe and understand issues related to adherence. Children in the study were asked to provide strategies for improving adherence. Strategies identified by the children for improving adherence included reminders from parents, social strategies such as taking medications in private, enhancing accessibility of the medications by placing them near their alarm clock, accepting responsibility for taking their own medications, and increasing their own motivation by recognizing the consequences of not taking medications, such as an increase in symptoms. Surprisingly, many children in the study admitted that nagging from parents was often a successful strategy for getting them to take their medications. After being asked to generate strategies to improve adherence, children were presented with specific strategies posed by the moderator based on behavioral theory. Behavioral concepts endorsed by the children included reinforcement contingencies such as receiving rewards for taking their medications, stimulus control strategies such as the use of alarms to help them remember, self-monitoring techniques such as using charts to keep track of their medications, modeling such as meeting with other children who have asthma in a group setting, and problem-solving strategies such as meeting with an asthma coach or mental health professional. Reinforcement contingencies were the most frequently endorsed strategies by the children.[4] Other strategies for enhancing adherence to therapy can be found in Table 47-1.[1,5]

The concept endorsed by the National Asthma Education and Prevention Program *Expert Panel Report 3: Guidelines for the Diagnosis and Management of Asthma* for creating an active partnership with the child and family can also positively affect adherence. Establishing a trusting patient-provider relationship through the use of open communication is one aspect of the partnership model that can help address nonadherence.

Table 47-1
Strategies for Increasing Adherence

- Open communication
- Reminder systems
- Reward systems
- Education regarding disease process and medication benefits
- Common goal setting
- Identifying barriers to adherence
- Routine follow-up including phone follow-up
- Simplifying treatment plan (ie, daily or twice daily dosing, same type of delivery device)
- Provide patient with samples, coupons, and resources for medication assistance programs
- Referral to psychologist/psychiatrist as indicated
- Instituting visiting nurse services
- Encourage patient to enlist the support of family members
- Provide culturally appropriate written educational materials that are written no higher than a fifth-grade reading level

Identifying and addressing patient and family concerns about asthma care and treatment can help target both volitional and inadvertent forms of nonadherence. Finally, identifying patient and parent treatment preferences and developing goals together while considering cultural beliefs will help address volitional forms of nonadherence.

References

1. Matsui D. Current issues in pediatric medication adherence. *Paediatr Drugs.* 2007;9:283-288.
2. Adams CD, Dreyer ML, Dinakar C, Portnoy JM. Pediatric asthma: a look at adherence from the patient and family perspective. *Curr Allergy Asthma Rep.* 2004;4:425-432.
3. Bender BG, Bender SE. Patient-identified barriers to asthma treatment adherence: responses to interviews, focus group, and questionnaires. *Immunol Allergy Clin North Am.* 2005;25:107-130.
4. Penza-Clyve SM, Mansell C, McQuaid EL. Why don't children take their asthma medications? A qualitative analysis of children's perspectives on adherence. *J Asthma.* 2004;41:189-197.
5. George M, Apter AJ. Improving adherence to asthma medications. *Clin Pulmon Med.* 2001;8:257-264.

ARE THERE PARTICULAR ASTHMA OUTCOMES OR QUALITY INDICATORS OF WHICH I NEED TO BE AWARE?

Gabriela Ramirez-Garnica, PhD, MPH

Children's health care quality measurement and improvement has attracted growing attention during the past decade.[1] Although a framework for the assessment of quality in health care was first presented by Donabedian in his classic 1966 paper,[2,3] until recently, little evidence was available about the quality of care delivered to children. Recent research points to deficiencies in the quality of ambulatory care delivered to children, and it has been reported that they receive only 46.5% of the indicated care.[4] Given that asthma is a common condition in children and is the cause of significant disability,[5,6] early efforts of assessing the pediatric health care quality included performance indicators of asthma care. However, to date, there have been few widely accepted performance metrics.

Asthma Is a Common Childhood Condition, and Its Burden Is Great

Current asthma prevalence rates among children aged 0 to 17 years are at historically high rates and continue to increase.[6] In 2007, 9.1% of children had asthma,[6] and by 2009, this rate had increased to 9.6%, affecting 7.1 million children.[7] Children with asthma can experience adverse outcomes, such as limitations in their daily activities, visits to the emergency department, and, although infrequent, death. For example, it has been reported that 40% of children with disabling asthma experienced a limitation in school attendance or were unable to attend.[5] The burden placed on the health care system by the large number of children with asthma has increased over time, and these children consume significant health care services. In 2007, children made 6.7 and 1.4 million visits to private physician offices and hospital outpatient departments, respectively. Further, 0.64 million emergency department visits were made and 157,000 hospitalizations.[7]

Guidelines for the Assessment and Management of Asthma Exist, but Some Gaps in the Quality of Asthma Care Have Been Identified

Although our understanding of the primary causes of asthma is imperfect, evidence-based guidelines for its treatment and management are available,[8] and the means for controlling and preventing symptoms are well-established.[7] In the third and most recent report, *Expert Panel Report 3* (EPR-3): *Guidelines for the Diagnosis and Management of Asthma* released in August 2007, 4 key components of care were identified: assessment and monitoring, education for a patient/provider partnership, control of environmental factors, and medications. To facilitate the use of the guidelines in clinical practice and to promote quality in asthma care, the Guidelines Implementation Panel (GIP) released a later report articulating 6 key clinical practice recommendations that correlated with the four components mentioned above (Table 48-1).[9]

Despite the large asthma burden and the existence of effective disease-control strategies, there are data pointing to a need for progress in key areas of asthma management. Using a composite quality indicator that measured 17 elements of asthma care, in one study, only 45.5% of children with asthma received the indicated care.[10] In another based on data from the National Health Interview Survey, only 44.3% and 53.2% of children were given an asthma management plan and advised to change things at home or school to improve asthma.[7] In a study assessing adherence to the National Heart, Lung, Blood Institute guidelines among primary-care providers, several negative practices, such as the use of cough suppressants and albuterol suspension, were identified.[11]

Measuring and Assessing the Quality of Pediatric Care

There are several definitions for quality. The term *quality* is generally used in the medical care literature to denote the extent to which a service or treatment, of known effectiveness, has been applied in accordance with accepted professional standards or targets.[12] The Institute of Medicine defined quality as the degree to which health services for individuals and population increase the likelihood of desired health outcomes and are consistent with current professional knowledge. Regardless of the definition used, the assessment of quality is an important activity in health care as it can serve to inform health care consumers, inform and determine payment and compensation decisions, drive improvement, and, most recently, support physician accreditation. For example, assessing and demonstrating quality has begun to impact physician credentialing.[1] The American Board of Medical Specialties (ABMS) requires engagement in quality improvement projects and the use of metrics for maintenance of certification (MOC). The recent passage of the Children's Health Insurance Program (CHIP) Reauthorization Act calls for the development of quality of care performance metrics to assess the care provided to children under this program.[13]

Donabedian conceptualized the most frequently used framework for measuring aspects of health care quality by defining 3 key domains related to the scope of inquiry:

Table 48-1

Summary of *Expert Panel Report-3* Care Components and Key Messages

Care Component	*Practice Recommendation*
Medications	Inhaled corticosteroids: Inhaled corticosteroids are the most effective medications for long-term management of persistent asthma and should be used by patients and clinicians as is recommended in the guidelines for control of asthma.
Education	Asthma action plan: All people who have asthma should receive a written asthma action plan to guide their self-management efforts.
Assessment and monitoring	Asthma severity: All patients should have an initial severity assessment based on measures of current impairment and future risk in order to determine type and level of initial therapy needed. Asthma control: At planned follow-up visits, asthma patients should review level of control with their health care provider based on multiple measures of current impairment and future risk in order to guide clinician decisions to either maintain or adjust therapy. Follow-up visits: Patients who have asthma should be scheduled for planned follow-up visits at periodic intervals in order to assess their asthma control and modify treatment if needed.
Control of environmental triggers	Allergen and irritant exposure control: Clinicians should review each patient's exposure to allergens and irritants and provide a multipronged strategy to reduce exposure to those allergens and irritants to which a patient is sensitive and exposed (ie, that make the patient's asthma worse).

structure, process, and outcomes.[2,3] Structure is defined as the conditions under which care is delivered. Process refers to the activities that constitute health care. Outcomes are the changes attributable to health care. In 1998, Mangione-Smith and colleagues proposed a conceptual framework for evaluating the quality of health care for the general population of children.[14] In later work, a 3-dimensional taxonomy of quality focused on type of care, function of medicine, and modality was proposed.[15] Type of care can be classified as acute, chronic, or preventive. The function of care was classified in 4 categories: screening, diagnosis, treatment, or follow-up. The modality of care was defined as the mechanisms through which screening, diagnosis, treatment, and follow-up are provided for preventive, acute, and chronic care. They include history, physical examination, laboratory, radiology, medication, counseling, referrals, and so on. In 2001, the Committee on Quality of Health Care in America proposed a focus on the following 5 aims for improving quality: safety, effectiveness, patient centeredness, timeliness, and equity.[16]

Using Donabedian's framework, quality metrics to assess the type, function, and modality of care can be developed. Further, it is also possible to assess how this care is reflective of the 6 properties of quality identified by the Institute of Medicine. In fully assessing the quality of health care, having a set of comprehensive measures that assess structure, process, and outcomes would be ideal. However, most quality improvement efforts focus on process and outcomes measures. This is because data to assess processes are more readily available and are available sooner. Assessing outcomes as measures of quality can be more difficult for several reasons. First, long periods of time may have to elapse before the outcome of interest is manifested. This is a particularly relevant limitation in pediatrics. Second, there have to be readily identifiable outcomes. Third, because many factors besides medical care influence outcomes, more sophisticated analytical methodology can be required.

A starting point for measure selection is the selection of the key quality questions to be assessed. Because developing valid and feasible measures can be difficult, using already established measures, if they exist, is more efficient. Validity in this case relates to whether there is adequate scientific evidence, or expert professional consensus, of the relationship between 1) structure and process, 2) structure and outcome, or 3) process or structure and outcome. A measure is considered feasible when the data needed for its calculation are available and these data sources are unbiased and free of random error.[13]

Currently Available Quality Measures of Pediatric Asthma Care

Quality assessments of the quality of care delivered to children with asthma have been included in several studies and have been the subject of quality initiatives.[7,10,11,17] In 2009, a comprehensive review of measures useful to assess the quality of state-level asthma care was published.[17] However, only a small number of these have been endorsed by the National Quality Forum (NQF).[18] The first core measure set specifically designed to evaluate the quality of care provided to hospitalized children was focused on processes of asthma care and includes 3 core measures.[19,20] However, these 3 measures only serve to assess processes delivered in a hospital setting and for the population of children admitted with an asthma exacerbation. Because much of the care delivered to these children is in the context of an outpatient setting and relates to other functions of care, several other metrics have been proposed and are in use by various organizations. In addition, an asthma care measure was recently developed for inclusion in the Medicaid and CHIP set of quality measures.[13,21] Using the EPR-3 care components as a framework, 8 process measures are listed (Table 48-2). Except for the EPR-3 care component of Control of Environmental Triggers, for which no NQF-endorsed quality measure exists, there is at least one measure for each of the other EPR-3 care components. Outcome measures are listed in Table 48-3.

Table 48-2

Process Measures Assessing the Quality of Asthma Care

EPR-3 Care Component	Measure	Definition	Type and Function of Care Being Assessed; Setting of Care
Assessment and monitoring	Asthma assessment	Percentage of patients who were evaluated during at least one office visit for the frequency (numeric) of daytime and nocturnal asthma symptoms	Chronic, diagnosis; clinician's office
Education	Home Management Plan of Care document given to patient/caregiver (CAC-3)	Documentation exists that the Home Management Plan of Care (HMPC) as a separate document, specific to the patient, was given to the patient/caregiver, prior to or upon discharge.	Acute, treatment; hospital
	Management plan for people with asthma	Percentage of patients for whom there is documentation that a written asthma management plan was provided either to the patient or the patient's caregiver or, at a minimum, specific written instructions on under what conditions the patient's doctor should be contacted or the patient should go to the emergency room.	Chronic, treatment; clinician's office
Medications	Use of appropriate medications for people with asthma	Percentage of patients who were identified as having persistent asthma during the measurement year and the year prior to the measurement year and who were dispensed a prescription for either an inhaled corticosteroid or acceptable alternative medication during the measurement year.	Chronic, treatment; clinician's office

(continued)

Table 48-2 (continued)

Process Measures Assessing the Quality of Asthma Care

EPR-3 Care Component	Measure	Definition	Type and Function of Care Being Assessed; Setting of Care
Medications (continued)	Use of relievers for inpatient asthma (CAC-1)	Percentage of pediatric asthma inpatients, age 2 to 17, who were discharged with a principal diagnosis of asthma who received relievers for inpatient asthma.	Acute, treatment; hospital
	Use of systemic corticosteroids for inpatient asthma (CAC-2)	Percentage of pediatric asthma inpatients (age 2 to 17 years) who were discharged with a principal diagnosis of asthma who received systemic corticosteroids for inpatient asthma.	Acute, treatment; hospital
	Pharmacologic therapy	Percentage of all patients with mild, moderate, or severe persistent asthma who were prescribed either the preferred long-term control medication (inhaled corticosteroid) or an acceptable alternative treatment.	Chronic, treatment; clinician's office
	Use of short-acting beta-agonist inhaler for rescue therapy	Percentage of patients with asthma who have a refill for a short-acting beta-agonist in the past 24 months.	Chronic, treatment; clinician's office

More work is needed to further the development of asthma performance metrics to assess the multiple dimensions of quality for asthma care. There is evidence of improved performance in important core areas of asthma care. For example, according to data from the National Committee for Quality Assurance, the percentage of commercial members identified as having persistent asthma who were prescribed recommended medications has improved from 57.7% in 1999 to 92.7%. Among Medicaid, the rate has improved from 60.1% in 2001 to 88.6% by 2009.[22] However, research is also needed to further assess the usefulness of existing metrics and also the purported relationships between processes and outcomes. In a recently published evaluation of hospital-level compliance with the

Table 48-3

Outcomes Measures Assessing the Quality of Asthma Care

Measure	Definition	Type and Function of Care Being Assessed; Setting of Care
Pediatric asthma admission rate	Admission rate for asthma in children ages 2 to 17, per 100,000 population (area level rate)	Acute; other
Pediatric asthma-related emergency room visit rate	Asthma emergency department use for all children 2 through 20 years of age diagnosed with asthma or treatment with at least two short-acting beta-adrenergic agents during the measurement year with one or more asthma-related emergency department visits.	Acute; emergency room
Asthma emergency department visits	Percentage of patients with asthma who have greater than or equal to one visit to the emergency room for asthma during the measurement period.	Acute; hospital

3 asthma pediatric core measures, researchers found high compliance with appropriate prescription of appropriate medications during admission for children admitted with an asthma exacerbation, and whether these metrics are useful has been called into question.[20] This same study found moderate hospital adherence with CAC-3 (being discharged with a home management plan of care) and subsequent emergency department visits and asthma-related re-admissions. Similar evaluations are needed to assess the usefulness of existing process measures for the outpatient setting.

Summary

Pediatric asthma is an area of medicine that lends itself well to the measurement of quality care. The implementation of quality metrics in the management of pediatric asthma can be done efficiently and in an evidence-based manner. Electronic medical records further facilitate this process, which can enhance patient outcomes in important ways by ascertaining that patients are receiving the appropriate therapies and defining relevant gaps in care. Implementation of quality metrics and process improvement strategies is also becoming integrated with the concept of continuous professional development, and they can serve as markers for physician performance. The measurement of quality indicators in medical practice is here to stay, and pediatric asthma is a robust model for this process.

References

1. Werk LN, Milov DE, Lawless ST. A win-win scenario—using the electronic health record to facilitate quality improvement and achieve physician maintenance of certification. *JHIM*. 2011;25:32-40.
2. Donabedian A. The quality of medical care. *The Milbank Quarterly*. 2005;83:691-729.
3. Donabedian A. *An Introduction to Quality Assurance in Health Care*. Oxford, England: Oxford University Press; 2003.
4. Mangione-Smith R, DeCristofaro AH, Setodji CM, et al. The quality of ambulatory care delivered to children in the United States. *N Engl J Med*. 2007;357:1515-1523.
5. Newacheck PW, Halfon N. Prevalence, impact, and trends in childhood disability due to asthma. *Arch Pediatr Adolesc Med*. 2000;154:287-293.
6. Akinbami LJ, Moorman JE, Garbe PL, Sondik EJ. Status of childhood asthma in the United States, 1980-2007. *Pediatrics*. 2009;123:S131-S145.
7. Akinbami LJ, Moorman JE, Liu X. Asthma prevalence, health care use and mortality: United States, 2005-2009. *National Health Statistics Reports Number 32*. Retrieved from www.cdc.gov/nchs/data/nhsr/nhsr032.pdf. Published on January 12, 2011. Accessed March 15, 2011.
8. National Asthma Education and Prevention Program. *Expert panel report 3 (EPR-3): guidelines for the diagnosis and management of asthma*. Bethesda, MD: National Heart, Lung, and Blood Institute, 2007. NIH publication no. 08-4051.
9. National Heart, Lung, and Blood Institute. *Guidelines implementation panel report for expert panel report 3: guidelines for the diagnosis and management of asthma. Partners putting guidelines into action*. Bethesda, MD: National Heart, Lung, and Blood Institute, 2008. NIH publication no. 09-6147.
10. Mangione-Smith R, DeCristorfaro AH, Setodi CM, et al. The quality of ambulatory care delivered to children in the United States. *N Engl J Med*. 2007;357:28-52.
11. Rastogi D, Shetty A, Neugebauer R, Harijith A. National Heart, Lung, and Blood Institute guidelines and asthma management practices among inner-city pediatric primary care providers. *Chest*. 2006;129:619-623.
12. Macbeth HM. *Health Outcomes: Biological, Social and Economic Perspectives*. Oxford, England: Oxford University Press; 1996.
13. Mangione-Smith R, Schiff J, Dougherty D. Identifying children's health care quality measures for Medicaid and CHIP: an evidence-informed, publicly transparent expert process. *Academic Pediatrics*. 2011;11(suppl 3): 11-21.
14. Mangione-Smith R, McGlynn EA. Assessing the quality of healthcare provided to children. *HSR: Health Services Research*. October 1998. Part II, 33:4, 1059-1090.
15. McGlynn EA, Mangione-Smith R, Adams J. The quality of ambulatory care delivered to children in the United States [technical appendix]. *N Engl J Med*. 2007;357:28-52.
16. Institute of Medicine. *Crossing the Quality Chasm: A New Health System for the 21st Century*. Washington, DC: National Academy Press; 2001.
17. Agency for Healthcare Research and Quality. *Asthma care quality improvement: a resource guide for state action*. Retrieved from www.ahrq.gov/qual/asthmacare/. AHRQ Publication no. 06(09)-0012. Published September 2009. Accessed November 12, 2009.
18. National Quality Forum. *NQF-endorsed standards*. Retrieved from www.qualityforum.org/Measures_List.asp x?keyword=asthma&from=header#p=1&k=pediatric%2520asthma&e=1&st=&sd=&s=. Accessed May 15, 2011.
19. National Association of Children's Hospitals and Related Institutions. *Children's asthma care (CAC) core measure set background*. Retrieved from www.childrenshospitals.net/AM/Template.cfm?Section=Search3&template=/CM/HTMLDisplay.cfm&ContentID=43665. Accessed March 15, 2011.
20. Morse RB, Hall M, Fieldston ES, et al. Hospital-level compliance with asthma care quality measures at children's hospitals and subsequent asthma-related outcomes. *JAMA*. 2011;306:1454-1460.
21. Centers for Medicare & Medicaid Services; Center for Medicaid; CHIP and Survey & Certification; Children and Adults Health Programs Group. *CHIPRA Initial Core Set Technical Specifications Manual 2011*. Retrieved from www.cms.gov/MedicaidCHIPQualPrac/Downloads/CHIPRACoreSetTechManual.pdf. Published February 2011. Accessed October 5, 2011.
22. National Committee for Quality Assurance. *The State of Health Care Quality: Reform, the Quality Agenda and Resource Use*. Washington, DC: NCQA; 2010.

WHICH OF MY PATIENTS WITH ASTHMA SHOULD SEE A SUBSPECIALIST?

Aaron S. Chidekel, MD

While asthma remains the most common chronic disease of childhood and a condition that primary-care practitioners should be comfortable managing, there will be times when subspecialty evaluation is necessary or requested by a concerned family. The common situations for which subspecialty referrals for asthma are recommended are well-defined in asthma guidelines (Table 49-1). These recommendations are generally supported by outcomes studies demonstrating improvements in parameters, such as decreased emergency department visits or hospitalizations, as well as improvements in asthma-related symptoms and health-care costs. Subspecialty-guided care programs for pediatric asthma have been most successful when they have included ongoing follow-up, asthma education, and the provision of a clear action plan.

In general, the need for consultation with a subspecialist can be considered in alignment with the asthma guidelines themselves: Referral can occur due to excessive or persistent patient impairment. Referral may be needed due to the risk of an adverse asthma outcome. A patient may need further evaluation for asthma comorbidities or exacerbating environmental factors. An additional reason for referral may be the need for more intensive education than can be provided in a primary-care setting. Finally, the patient may require complex medical management that can be more readily facilitated by an asthma specialist.

Excessive asthma impairment and risk are closely linked and together represent poorly controlled asthma. Those children in whom symptoms are severe, persistent, or atypical are all candidates for subspecialty referral. Asthma guidelines specifically suggest that patients with frequent and/or severe exacerbations, including those with a history of hospitalization and frequent emergency department visits, those with a history of an intensive care unit admission or episode of respiratory failure, and children who have required more than 2 bursts of oral steroids in the past year, be evaluated

---

Table 49-1

Potential Reasons to Seek Subspecialty Referral for Asthma Impairment and Risk

- Risk
  - Life-threatening asthma
  - Recurrent hospitalization or emergency department visits
  - Frequent steroid use
  - Steroid dependence
  - Severe or atypical symptoms
  - *Expert Panel Report 3:* Steps 3 and 4 level care or higher (age 5 years and up)
  - *Expert Panel Report 3:* Steps 2 and 3 level care or higher (age 0 to 4 years)
- Evaluation for comorbidity or environmental triggers
  - Suspicion for an underlying condition is high
  - Presence of a significant comorbidity
  - Need for specialized testing
  - Consideration for immunotherapy
- Complex medical regimens
  - Need for multiple controller medications
  - Inadequate response to initial therapy
- Educational needs
  - Overt adherence problems
  - Need for intensive or specific asthma education
- Other
  - High-risk social situations

---

by an asthma specialist. An additional recommendation involves those children with persistent asthma requiring more intensive and complex asthma therapy (*Expert Panel Report 3* Steps 3 and 4 for older children and *Expert Panel Report 3* Steps 2 and 3 for children aged 0 to 4 years).

Patients with asthma should undergo evaluation for comorbidities or exacerbating environmental factors, and this may require subspecialty testing or care coordination. This evaluation may even require the services of different types of specialists if a child has multiple comorbidities. While most patients with asthma require minimal and straightforward testing, some will require testing that necessitates subspecialty evaluation. Detailed allergy testing for environmental triggers or food allergy is the most obvious example and is most frequently performed by an asthma-allergy specialist. Occasionally, other specialized tests, such as flexible bronchoscopy, exercise testing with or without laryngoscopy, exercise or other pulmonary challenge testing, or even polysomnography, will require referral to a pediatric pulmonologist. Other specialized testing or clinical evaluation might require the input of a gastroenterologist (symptomatic gastroesophageal reflux or eosinophilic esophagitis), an otolaryngologist (severe sinus disease), or an immunologist.

Prioritizing the differential diagnosis and tailoring the consult question(s) to the needs of the patient is important. So is trying to avoid the need for multiple visits to multiple specialists, each of whom will have their own biases and points of emphasis. This can quickly result in confusion for the patient if the evaluation or recommendations become fragmented or even contradictory. Clearly, there needs to be a physician who serves as the main point of contact to provide guidance and synthesis of the plan for the patient and family. It is also critical to define which physician is responsible for ordering and following up on the necessary tests. An important result can be overlooked or a test not ordered if it is unclear who is responsible for ensuring test completion and communication of the results with the family.

Patients who require complex medical regimens or intensive education are also candidates for subspecialty referral. Subspecialty practices may have resources for patient education that are simply unavailable in primary care. For example, in our pediatric pulmonology practice, we have respiratory therapists in clinic who regularly perform spirometry or review asthma devices and medication delivery systems. We also have nurse practitioners who can review other important aspects of asthma care, such as which medications should be taken and their purposes, environmental control interventions, and the implementation of an individualized asthma action plan. Other practices may have certified asthma educators or even offer specific asthma classes for patients.

Similarly, subspecialty physicians can assist in the management of children who require multiple medications. While the specialist will not have a "silver bullet" or other cure-all, they can provide input to the plan and help with medication titration and adjustment. If a patient is a candidate for allergen immunotherapy or omalizumab injections, this can be facilitated by the involvement of a subspecialist, most often an asthma-allergy physician.

When implementing a plan for subspecialty referral, there are several scenarios to consider and clarify. One scenario involves the consultant becoming responsible for the ongoing management of the patient as the primary asthma physician. Another scenario involves a one-time visit to the asthma specialist for evaluation and implementation or continuation of a previously established management plan. In this case, the primary care physician will remain the primary asthma physician. The third scenario involves the co-management of a child with asthma between the primary-care and subspecialty physician. In this case, the visits rotate between the physicians so that ongoing follow-up is adequately spaced with both physicians partnering in the care of the patient.

My personal experience is that each of these scenarios can be implemented successfully as long as communication is clear and expectations are established at the outset. For example, I might take over the asthma management of certain asthma patients, such as those with severe disease or complex respiratory comorbidities, whereas at other times, I will provide a one-time consult with recommendations about any additional testing and changes in therapy for an individual patient that are then implemented by the primary-care physician. Most often, the model employed in our community is one of collaborative co-management. However, this will vary from community to community and with other factors, such as the severity and complexity of the individual patient, the level of availability of subspecialists, and the level of comfort of primary-care physicians in managing asthma. Whatever the case, it is important for consultants and referring physicians to work collaboratively and with clarity so that the patient knows who to call and when to call and is not confused by conflicting messages or frustrated by a lack of access.

The asthma guidelines are fairly clear on which pediatric patients are good candidates for referral to an asthma specialist, most often a pediatric pulmonologist or asthma-allergy physician. The specialist can assume a primary role in asthma management or complement the management provided by a general pediatrician or family practice physician. This collaboration between family, primary care, and subspecialty physician can be rewarding and can successfully improve asthma outcomes as long as the overarching goal is to work collaboratively in a patient-centered fashion to enhance access and quality of care for the patient and to ease the overall burden of asthma on the family.

Suggested Readings

Bush A, Saglani S. Management of severe asthma in children. *Lancet*. 2010;376:814-825.

Fanta CH, Carter EL, Stieb ES, Haver KE. *The Asthma Educator's Handbook*. New York, NY: McGraw Hill Medical; 2007.

National Asthma Education and Prevention Program. *Expert panel report 3 (EPR-3): guidelines for the diagnosis and management of asthma*. Bethesda, MD: National Heart, Lung, and Blood Institute, 2007. NIH publication no. 08-4051.

Weinberger M. Seventeen years of asthma guidelines: why hasn't the outcome improved for children? *J Pediatr*. 2009;154:786-788.

FINANCIAL DISCLOSURES

Dr. Alia Bazzy-Asaad has no financial or proprietary interest in the materials presented herein.

Dr. Jonathan E. Bennett has no financial or proprietary interest in the materials presented herein.

Dr. Anita Bhandari has no financial or proprietary interest in the materials presented herein.

Dr. Brad Bley has no financial or proprietary interest in the materials presented herein.

Dr. Aaron S. Chidekel has no financial or proprietary interest in the materials presented herein.

Dr. Lisa Forbes has not disclosed any relevant financial relationships.

Dr. David E. Gellar has not disclosed any relevant financial relationships.

Dr. Gabriel G. Haddad has no financial or proprietary interest in the materials presented herein.

Dr. Natalie M. Hayes has no financial or proprietary interest in the materials presented herein.

Dr. Robert A. Heinle has no financial or proprietary interest in the materials presented herein.

Dr. Katherine A. King has no financial or proprietary interest in the materials presented herein.

Dr. Joel D. Klein has no financial or proprietary interest in the materials presented herein.

Dr. Jennifer LeComte has not disclosed any relevant financial relationships.

Dr. Holger Link has no financial or proprietary interest in the materials presented herein.

Dr. Stephen J. McGeady has not disclosed any relevant financial relationships.

Dr. Sheela Raikar has no financial or proprietary interest in the materials presented herein.

Dr. Gabriela Ramirez has not disclosed any relevant financial relationships.

Dr. Amy Renwick no financial or proprietary interest in the materials presented herein.

Dr. Julie Ryu has no financial or proprietary interest in the materials presented herein.

Dr. Jonathan M. Spergel has no financial or proprietary interest in the materials presented herein.

Dr. Concettina (Tina) Tolomeo is an Editor for the *Journal of Asthma and Allergy Educator* (SAGE Publications) and a Content Expert for an online asthma education program sponsored by Welltok, Inc.

Dr. Daniel J. Weiner has no financial or proprietary interest in the materials presented herein.

Dr. Lisa B. Zaoutis has no financial or proprietary interest in the materials presented herein.

INDEX

alternative therapies, 65–68
American Academy of Allergy, Asthma, and Immunology, 202
American College of Allergy, Asthma, and Immunology, 202
American Lung Association, 202
anatomic airway abnormality, 189
anomalous coronary artery, 158
anti-IgE monoclonal antibody therapy, 52
antibiotics, 9, 188
anticholinergic bronchodilators, 52
anticholinergics, inhaled, 187
apnea, infants, 174
arformoterol, 75
aspiration, 37, 132
assessment quality indicators, 242
Association of Asthma Educators, 202
Asthma and Allergy Foundation of America, 202
atopy, 19
atypical pneumonia, causes of, 94
ayruveda, 66

bacterial disease, recurrent, 220
bacterial infections, 220
bacterial pneumonia, recurrent, 220
barky cough, 37
barriers to adherence, 239
beclomethasone, 75
benign thymic hyperplasia, 36
    infants, 36
beta agonists, 52, 54–55, 184–186
biologically-based therapies, 66
bocavirus, 90
Bordetella pertussis, 94
breast feeding, 174
breathing exercises, 66
bronchiolitis, 189
    risk factors, 174
    symptoms of, 174
bronchiolitis obliterans, 36
bronchodilators, 53–54, 178
bronchomalacia, 36
bronchoprovocation testing, 159
bronchopulmonary dysplasia, 36, 132

bronchospasm
    exercise-induced, 160
    nocturnal, 126
bruising, 55
budesonide, 75
burden of asthma, 241

cardiac disease, 158
cardiomegaly, 36
cardiomyopathy, 158
cardiopulmonary disease, 174, 179
    chronic, 174
cardiopulmonary exercise testing, 159
Centers for Disease Control and Prevention, 202
central obesity, 55
chest physiotherapy, 188
chest wall disorders, 158
chest x-rays, 233–236
chiropractic, 66
chlamydia, 37, 189, 194
Chlamydia pneumoniae, 94, 189
Chlamydia psittaci, 94
chromones, 62
chronic asthma, 131–135
chronic cardiopulmonary disease, 174
chronic outpatient medications, 179
chronic sinusitis, 36
ciclesonide, 75
ciliary dyskinesia, 132
clubbing, 37
Coccidiodes species, 94
cockroaches, 9
common goal setting, 239
comorbidity, 250
complementary medicine, domains of, 66
complex medical regiments, 250
congenital abnormalities
    airways (vascular rings/sling), 132
    lung, 132
congenital airway abnormalities, 37
congenital heart disease, 132, 158
congestive heart failure, 36, 189
conjunctivitis, 37
consult via telephone, 141–144
continuous inhaled bronchodilators, 178

Printed in the United States
by Baker & Taylor Publisher Services